STRENGTH
AFTER 40

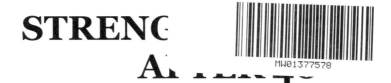

*How to Get and Stay in Shape.
A Step-by-Step Guide
(2022 Crash Course for Beginners)*

Cade Pearson

TABLE OF CONTENT

TABLE OF CONTENT i

INTRODUCTION... ii

OVERVIEW OF THE CHAPTERS viii

AUTHOR BIOGRAPHY xii

CHAPTER 1...1

   Your Body Has Changed 1

CHAPTER 2...18

Muscle Building at 40, 50, and Beyond 18

CHAPTER 3...32

   How Much Should You Lift? 32

CHAPTER 4...52

   Exercise Routines and Recovery Techniques............................52

CHAPTER 5...66

   Metabolism, Motivation, and Dedication 66

CHAPTER 6...79

   Eating Well, (and Loving It)...79

CHAPTER 7...100

   Common Fitness After 40 Misconceptions 100

CONCLUSION 103

INTRODUCTION

If you are over 40 and are determined to get into shape, whether for the first time or to regain your youthful physical condition, you have taken a crucial first step: This book's goal is to assist you.

achieve a stronger, leaner physique that leads to improved health and well-being, and to do so safely and effectively through exercise habits and lifestyle changes that are simple to adopt and implement

You are correct in your desire to construct a strong, lean physique by exchanging fat for muscle mass, increasing strength and endurance, enhancing your health, and raising your disease resistance. People over 40 can become strong and fit, but the workout routines that will bring them there will be different from when they were 20 or 25. Your body has changed, but with the right, scientifically evolved, and tried-and-true training strategies, you'll be astonished at how quickly you'll see and feel actual progress.

You'll be surprised how many people over 40 who were unhappy with their bodies and physical conditions decided to commit to getting in shape, doing it right, and getting the desired results. Building lean muscle mass, getting more definition, losing fat, especially around the belly, boosting energy and stamina, and feeling better about themselves are all beneficial outcomes. It may help you since your mental condition will improve with increased self-esteem, decreased anxiety, and a positive mindset that everything is possible regardless of your age.

What Are Your Fitness Objectives?

Do you want to be proud of yourself when you look in the mirror and see muscles that have returned after being soft and hidden beneath a layer of flab? Or have you noticed that your potbelly has shrunk as your abs have gotten more defined? Are you one of the two-thirds of Americans who are overweight or obese and want to reduce weight as an investment in your general health and longevity?

Do you know that your cardiovascular health should be a priority now that you're over 40? Do you aware that heart disease becomes a risk as you get older? How can heart attacks and strokes be avoided with good exercise and nutrition approaches?

It's Your Choice: **Motivation and Commitment**

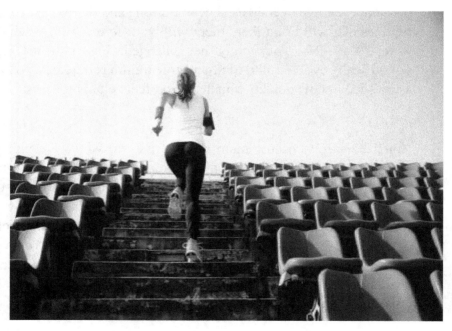

The degrees of your drive and commitment will determine whether you achieve your muscle- and strength-building goals and achieve true physical fitness. It's critical to remember that you'll be working out at least multiple times per week with resistance training that may include lifting, tugging, and stretching, as well as raising your heart rate for extended periods with cardio, or aerobic, workouts. Be confident that with the training suggestions you receive here, these workouts will not take up much time and are simple to learn.

Ask yourself why you want to get in shape and reach your fitness goals. What motivates you? There is no correct or incorrect reason for your commitment. What counts is that you have the motivation and determination to stick with it, beginning with the basic workouts and progressively progressing to more intense routines. You will not be alone in your decision to embrace the benefits of middle-age strength training.

Resistance workouts are available in fitness centers or your house Body calisthenics can be performed in a tiny, easy-to-assemble home gym. You can also do them without dumbbells.

Machines, barbells, and cables What matters most is your commitment to following the directions and performing the workouts, not the equipment. Don't become one of those folks that join a fitness center, buy equipment, and then never use it. Motivation and commitment are not the same as good intentions.

This is your road map.

This book will help you attain your fitness objectives. It understands the importance of presenting the most efficient training regimens for you while taking into account your age and current fitness level. Resistance and cardiovascular conditioning are clinically proven to be advantageous at any age, whether you are just turning 40 or long beyond. Furthermore, as you age, excellent dietary habits become increasingly important to your health and lifespan.

The motives that sparked your desire to begin a strengthening and conditioning program must be strong enough to keep you committed to making physical fitness and muscle-building an intrinsic part of your lifestyle. That is why we offer step-by-step training, options based on your particular tastes, and the freedom to exercise where and how you choose.

You Have the Opportunity

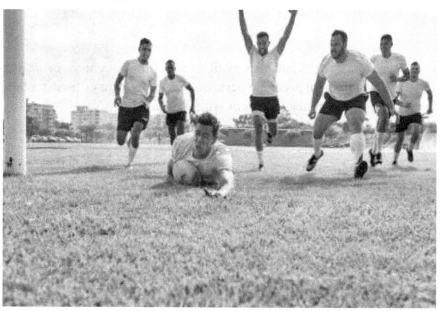

We hear the excuse "I don't have time to work out" all too often, and it can be uttered by men and women of any age.

The reality is that they are either unmotivated to begin an exercise routine or are strongly committed to maintaining it and incorporating it into their lives. They haven't realized how important their strength and fitness routines are for their health and wellness, as well as how they look and feel. To face those weights and cables, treadmill or exercise cycle at daybreak, before lunch or dinner, requires inner psychological power.

Nobody ever feels a good training session was a waste of time. On the contrary, they are pumped up by the satisfaction of correctly lifting weights, getting their heart rate up, and their arteries circulating, as well as the "high" that comes from the beta-endorphin chemicals released by hard exercise.

Exercises Designed for Your Age

This book was prepared for you at a point in your life when your physical health and overall fitness are no longer what they once were. The exercises you use to gain muscle and get in shape are not the same as they were when you were younger. We've done the research to determine which types of exercises and routines are ideal for you right now. You will discover how to get started, which exercises to do first, how frequently to train when to relax and recuperate, and how to progress. You will learn the core exercises to achieve the best results while avoiding complicated, sometimes hazardous workouts that are best left to professionals.

All of the strengthening exercises in this book are explained and demonstrated, so you won't have any trouble learning how to do them correctly.

Our workout requirements change as we age. Certain muscle groups require greater attention to maintain our bellies flat, protect our backs from soreness and suffering, enhance our balance, and prevent falls that can result in hip fractures and other serious injuries.

Weightlifting in middle age may necessitate a more cautious selection of weights, movements, repetitions, and rest times between sets. As you will see, hypertrophy, or the breaking down of muscle fibers and subsequent repair and rebuilding, lies at the heart of muscle building. Rest is critical to the success of this procedure. All of these aspects are taken into account in our training routines, so you don't have to.

OVERVIEW OF THE CHAPTERS

This book is designed to walk you through the characteristics of your body as you approach middle age. It will demonstrate that, even if your body has changed, you can still lift weights, use muscle-building equipment, and practice bodyweight calisthenics to build lean, well-defined muscle mass and grow stronger. You will be guided through cardiovascular workouts that you can do to improve your physical condition.

Your diet will play a vital role in your health and muscle-building efforts, and the guiding principles will serve as an incentive to get started and the determination to stick with it

Chapter 1 will help you understand how your body has grown and how it is not the same at 40 or older as it was at 20 or 25. Unless, of course, you've been working out with progressively larger weights consistently, which most of us haven't. The bulk of us have grown more sedentary, riding instead of walking or running, sitting instead of standing, and no longer lifting weights or performing calisthenics to keep our muscles tight and our bodies lean.

Our bodies have slowed as a result of our slowness, leaving us with less lean muscle mass and more body fat, as evidenced by an expanding waistline. This all adds up to you not being able to take up where you left off and do rigorous activities like you used to.

The second chapter will persuade you that your age does not impede accomplishing ambitious muscle-building goals. It's commonly known that you can build lean, muscular muscles after the age of 40.

It's simply a matter of executing the appropriate workouts with the appropriate weights and routines. Muscle and strength development requires the application of scientific and effective techniques that decrease the risk of damage while optimizing outcomes in the shortest amount of time. It is never too late to begin and now is a perfect moment to make the commitment and begin lifting.

Despite what you may have heard, Chapter 3 will reassure you of your ability to carry heavy weights. Being a middle-aged weightlifter does not imply that you can't lift high weights, or that heavier weights are only for kids, and you should lighten up.

Experience and research are not the same as opinions. Based on rigorous training and coaching, the research suggests that big weights are the way to go in middle age.

You will meet action-hero superstars whom you adore and who will discuss workouts that helped drive them to superstardom with you. If you want to create lean, well-defined muscle mass, heavier weights are the way to go as long as they aren't too heavy.

Chapter 4 discusses workout choices and recovery. You will be lifting large weights, but they will not be the same workouts you did when you were younger or that you see someone else doing at the fitness club. Some weightlifting exercises are appropriate for your age. Others that you may have done in the past are now too dangerous and should be avoided. Recovery time after intense activity was vital when you were younger to allow the hypertrophy rebuilding process to occur, but it's now doubly important because hypertrophy takes longer after age 40 and the risk of injury from overwork is higher. Your perseverance will be rewarded with fruition.

Chapter 5 is all about dedication. As your metabolism slows, the requirement for you to commit to physical fitness and muscle building is stronger. Each year, you lose more lean muscle mass as you get older. Simultaneously, your body increases its fat storage of surplus energy. That outcome is visible in your gut, and you ask, "Where did my six-pack abs go?" This is the time to examine yourself in the mirror and make the personal commitment to go the distance. Decide that no excuses will stop you from becoming a robust, strong, physically impressive person who tackles middle age with confidence.

The necessity of a healthy diet is discussed in Chapter 6. Your health, strength, and endurance are all affected by the fuel you consume, as well as the quality and variety of meals you consume. As important as weightlifting is for building muscle, becoming stronger, and being more fit, your diet is even more important. Carbohydrates, proteins, and fats in your diet should be sourced from nutritious, more natural, less processed foods that offer your body important vitamins, minerals, and antioxidants. There are numerous diets to choose from, but we'll introduce you to one that is more than simply a diet. It's a comprehensive lifestyle change that includes a wide variety of great foods that you'll enjoy without needing to calculate calories. We'll help you cut through all the nutritional misconceptions and embrace a lifelong dietary practice rather than a fad diet that will come and go by recognizing that our diet plays a crucial part in developing muscle and losing fat.

There are nutritional foundations that you will learn to follow.

Chapter 7 will discuss and dispel the myths that can undermine your dedication and motivation. You'll find that your workouts can be completed in less time than you expect.

That you may put forth actual effort and intensity in your fitness routines and get more out of your time and energy commitment.

You'll gain a new perspective on running, walking, and other proven types of cardiovascular fitness, and you'll grasp how food and exercise may work together to help you lose weight, boost your immune system, and prevent diseases.

CHAPTER 1

Your Body Has Changed

A new online article in WebMD (2020) emphasizes the necessity of exercise during middle age, arguing that while you no longer have the body of a 20-year-old, exercise that strengthens and gets you in shape is more vital now than when you were younger.

Being stronger and more physically fit is critical to preserving a good quality of life and independence as you grow older.

For those of us over 40, 50, or more, the benefits of weight training and other forms of resistance exercise, as well as keeping up aerobically with cardiovascular training, are significant.

Muscles burn more calories than body fat. Even when you're sleeping This can counteract the effects of middle-age metabolism slowing and make it easier to maintain a healthy weight.

pounds from piling up

Consistent exercise has been linked to a lower risk of developing life-threatening conditions in middle age, such as hypertension, strokes, atherosclerosis and other types of heart disease, diabetes, osteoporosis, and some types of cancer.

Strength and fitness training is thought to prevent the progression of Alzheimer's disease and other forms of dementia, as well as cognitive decline, which reduces the brain's sharpness.

These are the issues we'll examine in this chapter, and they'll help you understand, build up, and protect yourself.

"Know thyself," an old Greek aphorism, is etched as a maxim on the Temple of Apollo in Delphi, and it is a fitting prelude for your strength training after the age of 40. As you increase your enthusiasm and commitment, it is crucial to take a minute to reflect on who you are at this point in your life.

Because physical changes occur with age, your body is no longer that of a teenager or young adult. Some are caused by the natural wear and tear of life's stressors, while others are the product of the aging process. Your muscles are gradually atrophying, your ligaments, joints, and tendons are less flexible, and your resilience is slower, which means your recovery from severe exercise takes longer. Your body form may have shifted, and your belly may have expanded.

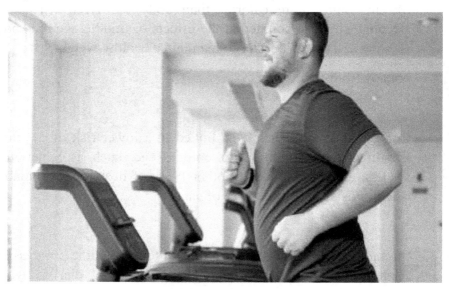

Other, more subtle alterations may be silently at work behind the scenes, slowing down your metabolism, or the general rate at which your body functions.

All of this adds up to you not being able to resume lifting weights and doing intensive workouts like you used to. However, it is not too late to resume a complete workout and fitness program centered on weightlifting.

Through exercise and diet, you can halt the aging process, repair lost muscle mass, create new, larger muscles, and gain significant strength. That is the focus of this book: recovering your body's previous strength, creating new muscle mass, increasing flexibility, losing weight, and keeping your arteries free to delay the start of cardiovascular disease.

Benchmarking 1: Taking Stock

Before beginning your weight training and overall physical improvement program, the best method to objectively identify where you are physically right now is to assess your current state. The first element of this benchmarking assessment is how you appear and compare to others.

The mirror, scale, and tape measure are all objective assessors of your progress and can help you create goals for where you want to go. Begin by staring in the mirror in your underwear and assessing your appearance objectively.

Don't be too hard on yourself; simply examine where you are currently and use it as a baseline, a starting point. Examine your upper arms: how solid and defined are the biceps in front and the triceps in back? Are your pectorals, sometimes known as "pecs," starting to sag? Next, do you have a definition for your

abdominal muscles or a sign of a well-developed "six-pack"? What about your thighs and calves? If you

Can you notice any definition in your legs if you stand sideways and lower yourself partially into a half-deep knee bend?

Make a mental note of what you observe, or better yet, write it down.

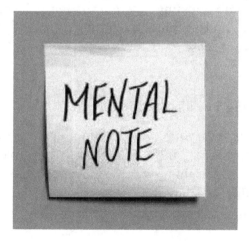

Step on the scale in your underwear, barefoot, and at the same time and condition every day, preferably before breakfast. After you've recorded your weight on the first day, go online and calculate your Body Mass Index (BMI), which is dependent on your height and weight. A BMI of 18.5 to 24.9 is regarded normal, 25 to 29.5 is considered overweight, and 30 or higher is considered obese. Don't be disappointed if you are overweight or obese; two-thirds of

American people are but commit to working to reduce their weight to a normal range. It is critical:

According to the National Heart, Lung, and Blood Institute (2020), the higher a person's BMI, the higher their risk of diseases like type 2 diabetes, heart disease, and high blood pressure.

High blood pressure, respiratory issues, gallstones, and some cancers

Be patient: just as it took time to develop the excess weight, it will take time to lose it. Along with exercise, your diet will play an important part, so pay close attention to the forthcoming chapter on diet.

The tape measure, like the scale, is fully objective in terms of appearance and physical measurement. It never lies, exaggerates, or coddles you.

Measure your waistline at the point where your hip bones meet your naval, pulling the tape firmly but not too tightly. Exhale right before measuring. Keep in mind that a man's measurement should not exceed 40 inches (102 cm), and a woman's measurement should not exceed 35 inches (89 cm).

Professionals claim that beyond such measurement limitations, there is too much belly fat, which can interfere with a variety of physical activities. It may also result in the same disorders as having a high BMI.

Measuring Strength in Benchmarking

The second element of your benchmarking assessment is to determine your level of strength. A certified personal trainer can take you through a series of measurements with various workouts and may even calculate your body fat and lean muscle percentages.

You can, however, take your simple strength measurement by bending down and counting how many push-ups you can perform.

Begin in a plank posture, with your legs stretched behind you, your arms fully extended shoulder-width apart, and your back level (no sagging or arching). Lower your head or chest to the floor, then raise back up to the beginning position and repeat as many times as you can. Don't rush: each down-and-up cycle should take roughly three seconds. Make a note of your total.

Count how many pull-ups you can complete with your hands facing forward if you have access to a pull-up or chin-up bar. Place your hands shoulder-width apart and pull up fully, then lower slowly ((not too quickly), and repeat as many times as you can in good form (no half-ways). When you're finished, make a note of the total. Alternatively, if you can use dumbbells, establish the greatest weight you can curl eight to ten times. A curl is performed by raising the dumbbells from the arms-lowered posture to your shoulders and then slowly lowering them back down.

As your weight training program improves, you can repeat these exercises regularly to track your development.

Longevity, Fitness, and Health

Your motivation to start or return to weightlifting and other workouts to increase strength in middle age is, at least in part, determined by how you want to appear and feel. You want to look in the mirror and see a well-built figure with obviously larger, defined muscles and a flatter stomach. At the end of your workouts, you want to feel the muscles expanding under your skin as blood rushes to the hard-working muscle cells and fibers in the "pumping iron" effect.

You want more energy, more bounce in your step, and more endurance to keep you going for a longer period. You wish to seem and feel fit. You want to be more powerful.

These are the motivators that will get you started on your weight-loss and muscle-building regimen. They should be enough to keep you going because reaching your fitness objectives will require time and work.

To reaffirm your commitment, let's return to what was said earlier in the benchmarking discussion: the health aspects of getting in shape and remaining in shape, as well as losing and maintaining weight.

Add Years to Your Life

There's an expression that originated with long-distance runners and has now expanded to weightlifting and fitness.

"Working out and staying in shape will add more life to your years and may even add more years to your life," says the community as a whole.

In other words, your devotion to muscle building and cardiovascular fitness will undoubtedly make every day richer and livelier, and may even help you live longer. Overall, it's not a horrible deal. It gives you something to work for, something to put time and energy into, and something to stick with in the long run.

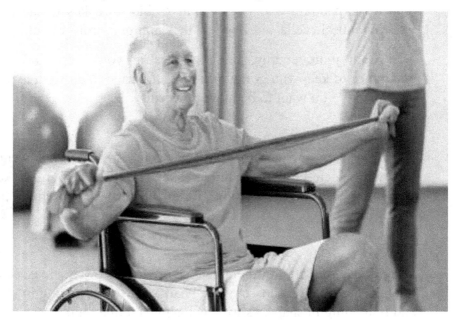

Regular exercise, according to the Mayo Clinic (2020), can enhance health and manage the symptoms of long-term chronic conditions that limit activities and interfere with normal living. Exercise is discussed individually in the next section due to its role in avoiding heart disease.

Everyday occurrences Weightlifting strength training not only improves muscle strength and endurance, but it also makes daily activities easier and reduces the reduction in muscle strength caused by disease. Every day, we lift, carry, stand, walk, squat, bend, and otherwise tax our muscles, joints, bones, and tendons, as well as our circulatory and respiratory systems when we strain our hearts and lungs during exercise. The higher our physical condition, the easier the work we do, and we feel better when we're in good shape.

Stability of the joints. Stability exercises can help you restore an optimal range of motion by giving stability to your joints and enhancing their functionality, and flexibility exercises can help you regain an optimal range of motion. When done correctly, weightlifting and other resistance exercises promote stability and flexibility while also strengthening the muscles that support the joints. By strengthening the quadriceps, for example.

We can help manage the kneecap and knee socket by using the muscles in the front of our thighs, preventing excessive motions that can wear away the cartilage that lubricates and cushions the knees.

Diabetes. Regular physical activity can reduce the incidence of adult-onset type 2 diabetes by allowing insulin to lower blood sugar levels.

levels more efficiently Resistance exercise with weightlifting, combined with aerobics, can minimize the risk of heart disease in people who already have type 2 diabetes.

Because type 2 diabetes is frequently connected with obesity, the weight-loss advantages of exercise can directly reduce diabetes risks and symptoms.

Weight management. Weightlifting and aerobic exercise both burn calories, so physical activity can help you regulate your weight and enhance your vitality. However, exercise \Salone does not optimize weight loss; it is the combination of diet \ and exercise that is most beneficial. In a later chapter, we'll look at how nutrition and exercise can work together to help you lose weight and keep it off for good.

Arthritis. Exercise has been shown to lower joint pain, maintain muscular strength in arthritis-affected joints, and reduce joint stiffness, resulting in improved quality of life and physical function in those who have had arthritis for years. Low-impact exercise is recommended for those suffering from arthritic symptoms. Any weightlifting that puts extra strain on joints may necessitate adjusting certain movements to decrease the strain.

Asthma. Weightlifting and other forms of intense exercise appear to help lower the severity and frequency of asthma attacks by requiring heavier, deeper breathing. The enhanced blood circulation and oxygen delivery, together with the depth of breathing during exercise, may strengthen the lungs and air sacs where oxygen is delivered to the bloodstream. Deep breathing during strenuous activity also helps to strengthen the

The diaphragm muscle regulates breathing by enabling inhalation and exhalation.

Backache. Resistance workouts that challenge your abdominal and core muscles to develop the muscles that surround your spine, and these

Exercises may help alleviate the symptoms of back discomfort. Low-impact aerobic workouts conducted regularly are also thought to be beneficial.

improve the function of the lumbar and thoracic back muscles and increase back strength and endurance Later, we'll go over stretching and flexibility routines that can help relieve your aching lower back in only a few minutes.

Bone mineral density. Our bones are naturally porous.

However, as we age, this porosity increases and the bones become less dense, brittle, and more prone to fracture. This is referred to as osteoporosis.

Falls are the most prevalent cause of bone fractures, but there are others, including some that are caused by activity.

Small stress fractures, which are hairline fissures in the bones that can cause pain and lead to larger breaks, can be caused by running or leaping on a hard surface, for example. However, the appropriate kind of exercise can help cure osteoporosis and strengthen bones:

Dancing, jumping rope, sprinting, and jogging outside (with correct athletic shoes to prevent injury), climbing (particularly uphill), and playing tennis or racquetball are all examples of high-impact, weight-bearing workouts.

Low-impact, weight-bearing exercises, such as working out on elliptical machines or stair climbers, and walking at a brisk moderate pace either outdoors or on a treadmill, may be healthier for people already diagnosed with osteoporosis.

Stretching and weightlifting using free weights, such as dumbbells and kettle weights, or weight machines with cable-pulled weights, are examples of muscle-strengthening activities.

Using elastic exercise bands or doing bodyweight calisthenics

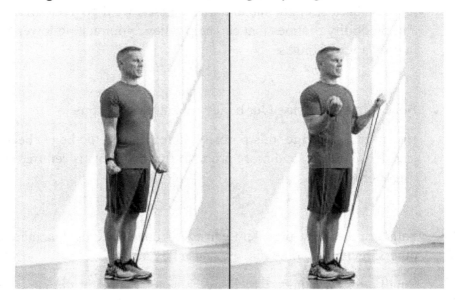

Stretching (particularly after a workout), yoga, and Pilates are all examples of flexibility exercises. Yoga has been shown to improve flexibility and balance, which can help reduce falls. If you already have osteoporosis issues, consult your doctor or a skilled professional physical therapist to ensure you are not overstretching body regions that are at risk.

Mental well-being. Exercise helps to alleviate the symptoms of two of the most frequent mental and emotional issues: anxiety and sadness. Both of these disorders are frequently the result of

Stress causes the body's sympathetic response, also known as the "fight or flight" response to perceived hazards. The human body prepares for action by increasing pulse and breathing rates and releasing energy chemicals such as adrenaline and cortisol Anxiety can develop in this charged condition, and if it persists over time or is chronic, it can lead to immunological reactions, including chronic inflammation.

Resistance or cardiovascular exercise capitalizes on the body's state of preparation by successfully putting energy hormones to work and burning the excess glycogen delivered to your muscles. When you finish your workout and cool down, your heart and breathing rates will return to normal. The workout will also cause the release of beta-endorphin chemicals, which will make you feel elated and relieve your worry.

Depression can arise when the parasympathetic nervous system overreacts, lowering typical energy levels and depressing the central nervous system. As with anxiety, beta-endorphin hormones can provide a sense of euphoria and lessen or eradicate the depressive state.

Caution: Chronic anxiety and depression may not react adequately to exercise, meditation, or yoga.

In some circumstances, professional assistance may be required.

Dementia. Exercise may help with cognition issues, especially in those with dementia. Furthermore, those who are not currently suffering from dementia and who engage in regular resistance and aerobic activities are at a lower risk of developing cognitive impairment and dementia or significantly reducing its onset.

Cancer. Can regular exercise help prevent cancer? According to the Mayo Clinic, there is evidence that exercise can reduce the risk of dying from prostate, breast, and colorectal cancer, and exercise may also help reduce the risk of getting other types of cancer. Exercise may help improve the quality of life and overall fitness of cancer survivors. Many experts feel that exercise's function in weight loss and lowering the risk of other diseases strengthens the immune system, which helps prevent cancer cells from proliferating, developing tumors, or metastasizing (spreading).

Cardiovascular Health

Exercise is closely associated with the prevention of heart disease, and for good reason. Exercise has been shown to help prevent or reduce the risk of heart disease.

Resistance and cardiovascular exercise, when conducted for a suitable amount of time and intensity, can enhance overall heart health and contribute to the prevention of heart attacks, heart failure, and strokes.

Atherosclerosis, or the build-up of plaque in the arteries, is a type of heart disease.

Plaque in the coronary arteries, which carry oxygen-rich blood to the heart. As the plaque builds up over time, the flow of

The flow of blood to the heart is constricted. Angina pectoris, or chest pain during exertion, is an early warning sign.

Controlling blood lipid levels is directly tied to preventing or minimizing plaque build-up.

Can exercising help you lose weight? Within limits, the findings of investigations are encouraging. HDL (good) cholesterol is attributed to transporting LDL (bad) cholesterol, the low-density, sponge-like blood lipid that can contribute to plaque that clogs arteries, leading to atherosclerosis or coronary heart disease.

Triglycerides, which are fats that circulate in the bloodstream and can also cause heart disease, are another significant blood lipid type.

Activity-induced decreases in LDL cholesterol and triglycerides, as well as increased beneficial HDL cholesterol, have been shown in studies, and the intensity of exercise is a critical role. Whether weightlifting or aerobics, the workout should raise the heart rate and sustain it there for at least 25 to 40 minutes three times each week.

Hypertension management. Exercise can also help to reduce hypertension, or high blood pressure, which is a leading cause of strokes.

Exercise and high blood pressure are linked because regular, consistent physical activity strengthens your heart. Your heart can pump more blood volume with less effort when it is stronger. As your heart works less to pump blood, your blood pressure falls as the pressure on your arteries decreases.

Exercise has been shown in studies to reduce systolic blood pressure (the first number in your blood pressure reading) by four to nine millimeters of mercury (mm Hg). So, with the correct exercise, a systolic pressure of 135 might be reduced to 126, which is within the normal range and similar to the effect of various blood pressure prescription medicines. As a result, for some people with hypertension, regular exercise might reduce or eliminate the need for blood pressure medication.

The benefits of exercise extend to persons with normal blood pressure (less than 130/80 mm Hg). Exercise can help prevent blood pressure from rising as you age. Another method of exercise that might help you control your blood pressure is by helping you maintain a healthy weight and BMI.

Resistance exercise has also been shown to benefit cardiovascular health. Researchers found in BMC Public Health (2012) that combining resistance and aerobic exercise was more beneficial than any of these exercise approaches alone in helping patients shed more weight and fat while also increasing overall cardiovascular fitness.

Resistance training's lipid-lowering advantages for persons with high total cholesterol were reported in the medical journal Atherosclerosis (2011), demonstrating that those who exercised eliminated LDL cholesterol from their system faster than those who did not.

High-intensity interval training is generally safe and beneficial for the majority of people, and it may be completed in less time. In high-intensity interval training, you alternate between high-intensity exercise and low-intensity exercise.

Exercise at a lower intensity for short periods. Even higher-intensity activities like walking count.

Low-intensity exercise is beneficial for weight loss and stress relief, and some studies suggest that even walking at a moderate speed for 150 minutes per week can have favorable cardiovascular and general health effects. This intensity and duration are an alternative to the commonly suggested 75 minutes of vigorous exercise each week.

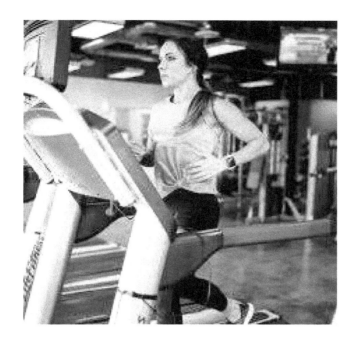

Post-coronary exercise is often recommended to promote healing and strengthen the heart, which is a muscle and, like all muscles, requires rest and recuperation. advantages of regular exercise the type and intensity of exercise should be medically supervised in these instances.

Let's go on to Chapter 2 and see what you can do.

Muscle building at 40, 50, and beyond

CHAPTER 2

Muscle Building at 40, 50, and Beyond

Do you have reservations? Do you believe that the years have passed you by and that you should have started weightlifting and bodybuilding ten, twenty, or more years ago? Or you used to lift weights but your career got in the way and you quit? Those years may have passed, but your chance to build those muscles and gain that power is still here, waiting for you to declare to yourself, "This is my moment to make up for lost time and build the body I've always wanted."

Consider Tug McGraw's admonition, "Yaa got to believe," which turned around the struggling New York Mets and propelled them to the 1974 World Series. It's all about thinking positively and believing in oneself.

It isn't too late. Even if you're in your forties and have never worked out, if you're overweight, out of shape, and out of energy, it's not too late. If you have the motivation and dedication to begin and maintain a weightlifting program, now is the time. If you are prepared, you can achieve your fitness, health, and energy goals. Yes, you can lift heavy weights and gain lean muscle mass. You've got this.

Science **The Muscle-Building**

To boost your confidence and dispel any doubts you may have about your ability to become a successful weightlifter at this point in your life, this chapter will provide you with the fundamentals from science and experience to convince you that there are physiological processes you can initiate that will reward you generously with results that will surprise, if not astound you.

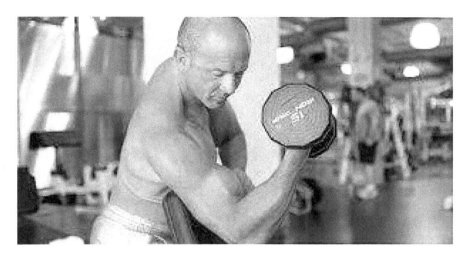

Science may not be the first thing that springs to mind when organizing a muscle-building program, but it is critical to disregard old clichés and anecdotal tales because creating lean muscles safely and effectively is fully founded on scientific principles. What exactly does this mean? According to the scientific method, facts are established by test results that can be reliably repeated, rather than by views and traditions. The same principles that apply to young weightlifters apply to middle-aged weightlifters, with the caveat that age necessitates some adaptations to obtain good results safely.

The Hypertrophy Concept

We're talking about the 650 skeletal muscles that allow us to move and accomplish work. They are composed of muscle fibers, which are composed of small thread-like fibers known as sarcomeres and myofibrils. These muscle fibers are the building blocks of muscular contraction. When you flex a muscle or put it to work, the activity takes place within the fibers. Keep these fibers in mind as we go since they will be the growth units that will strengthen and increase your muscles.

When specific nerves, known as motor neurons, receive messages from cells known as the sarcoplasmic reticulum, muscles contract on command. The signals will get more adept at getting your muscles to contract as your body grows more conditioned, and you will become stronger even before your muscles are substantially larger. If you can properly exercise to stimulate your motor neurons, you can jumpstart the processes of building bigger muscles to lift higher weights. This will be explained in greater depth in the instructional chapters.

First, cause harm. The process of hypertrophy, or muscle growth, begins with muscle fiber injury caused by weightlifting. The high effort of lifting or pushing big weights causes some of the muscle fibers involved in the hard exertion to break down; this happens at the cellular level and is natural. Your cells are being sacrificed because they are being asked to do more work than they are used to.

Repair the damage next. To repair the damage, cells employ amino acid molecules to fuse into muscle fibers and produce new myofibrils from protein strands. This is why protein is such a vital part of a weightlifter's diet; it is the building block from which myofibrils are made.

Importantly, during the hypertrophy process, the myofibrils are not only repaired and rebuilt to their original size, but they are also thicker and more numerous.

They get slightly bigger. They are developing.

When the muscles enlarge, they hypertrophy.

Muscle protein production has surpassed the pre-damage level. Muscle tissue is used daily.

The increments are small, but they add up with time, and muscle growth becomes evident.

Cells in orbit. The efficiency of your hypertrophy is dependent on satellite cells, which stimulate myofibril growth by boosting muscle protein nuclei and allowing the cells to divide more frequently. The degree to which satellite cells are active, according to trainer and coach John Leyva, technical editor of the Built Lean Blog (2020), is based on the type and resistance of the exercises performed, as well as the amount of stress exerted on the muscles:

1. Muscle tension is caused by gradually increasing the load that muscles are lifting and tugging, above the amount of resistance they are accustomed to. So, if you do bicep curls with 15-pound dumbbells regularly, your biceps and upper arms will preserve their current muscular size and strength but will not become larger or stronger unless you increase the weight to apply more resistance and stress.

2. Damage to muscle cells and tissues releases immune system cells and inflammatory chemicals, which activate satellite cells, which increase muscle tissue protein growth and boost hypertrophy. Muscle discomfort in the hours and even days following your workout is a strong indication that something has occurred. This is due to the damage done during the workout, and it lays the groundwork for the subsequent over-rebuilding of muscle tissue. Most of the soreness is due to lactic acid accumulation, which will go away in a day or two.

3. Metabolic stress is caused by severe muscle tension and results in the enlargement of the cells within and surrounding the muscle. It is the effect of blood accumulation that is causing this.

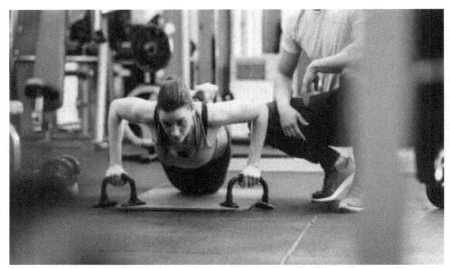

More oxygen to the tight and damaged muscle fibers, as well as the arrival of glycogen, the sugar molecules that provide energy to the muscle cells These effects, may contribute to increased rebuilding, but much of the increased muscle size after the workout is transitory, and the muscles will return to their regular size as the fluids drain from the muscles.

Hormones

The role of hormones in muscle growth is extensively contested. This is what we know about our body's natural hormones today:

The two most active hormones that contribute to muscle growth are testosterone and insulin-like growth factor I (IGH-I).

While testosterone levels are higher in males, women have testosterone (and men have estrogen), but a woman's testosterone is lower, which is one of the reasons why men may build muscles more easily than women.

Weightlifting and other resistance activities can help both men and women gain strength.

While the majority of our testosterone is not free-roaming or available to affect muscle building, studies show that high-intensity resistance exercise can increase testosterone levels, which can activate satellite cells, prevent or reduce protein breakdown, increase protein synthesis, and stimulate other anabolic hormones. It may also increase the sensitivity of muscle cell receptors to free testosterone. Testosterone can also boost growth hormone responses and increase the number of neurotransmitters at the site of a damaged fiber.

The bottom line regarding natural hormones in our bodies is that resistance training can trigger the production of hormones that further enhance muscle and strength gain.

Supplements for hormones? Hormone supplements to develop muscle growth are not recommended unless prescribed by a doctor after a blood test reveals a hormone deficiency.

Muscle Gain vs. Rest and Muscle Loss

The muscle repairs and rebuilding we've been describing don't happen while you're lifting weights and destroying your muscle fibers. Instead, muscle development (hypertrophy) occurs while you and your muscles are at rest.

Recovery can take place only during rest. If the muscles are continually pushed, even at less extreme levels, there will be little opportunity for hypertrophy to occur and, at best, no repairs will be possible. More importantly, strong resistance exercise performed too soon after a solid weightlifting session can have severe consequences:

If your muscles do not get enough rest to prepare,

By fixing them, you can reverse the protein-building process and allow your body to enter a dormant state.

catabolic or destructive state This can result in muscle atrophy over time.

After a resistance workout session, the time required for recuperation and hypertrophy is approximately 24 to 48 hours. Weightlifting that targets a certain muscle group should avoid working that muscle group for at least one day, ideally two.

If you conduct total-body resistance workouts in a single workout session, you should not do weightlifting or resistance sessions more than three times per week.

Over-40 weightlifters Rest and recuperation are especially important for you as a middle-aged weightlifter because your recovery period is longer due to your age and your slower metabolism. You should rest and recover for two days after each weightlifting exercise.

Increase your protein intake. During rest and recovery days, your diet should be high in protein since the amino acids that make up protein molecules are required for muscle fiber repair.

We'll go into the diet in further detail later, but for now, presume you'll want to consume more meat, fish, dairy, and eggs, all of which are high in complete protein.

Vegans and vegetarians can boost their intake of beans and other legumes, as well as soybeans, buckwheat, and quinoa, which are among the few plant sources of complete protein, including the nine necessary amino acids that our bodies require from our diet.

It's Not Too Late for People Over 40

We've just gone over the scientific foundation for muscle gain, and you can see there's no magic or mystery involved. Muscles can be built through resistance training, appropriate rest and recuperation, and a high-protein diet.

The cells that make up your muscles are broken, then repaired with protein, and the cells then over-repair.

As a result, your lean muscle tissue grows in size and strength over time. If the rules of the game are obeyed, hypertrophy is unavoidable.

Yes, you may think it works for the young, but you are over 40, 50, or 60, and you are now being taught that it is not too late for you to develop those muscles bigger and stronger.

How is this possible? Your muscles become smaller as you age, some body fat accumulates, your energy levels drop, and your knees, shoulders, and other joints pain when you bend, crouch, or lift something. Your testosterone level has decreased. Your bones' porosity may have increased, osteoporosis may be present, and your bones may be more prone to fracture.

A Perfect Moment

So, in conclusion, is it a good time to begin or resume heavy weightlifting and other forms of resistance exercise? Is it not too late?

As you have already read, it is not only not too late, but it is also a perfect time. Muscles that are bigger and stronger are not a sign of vanity.

They protect you from being weaker, frailer, more fragile, less mobile, less flexible, and, most importantly, less likely to be overweight or obese, putting you at risk for heart disease, diabetes, and a slew of other dangerous ailments. Right now, is your time. You have nothing to lose and everything to gain in terms of health, longevity, strength, energy, and vitality, a terrific build to be proud of, and self-esteem.

In his TC Nation (2019) article, weightlifting coach and trainer TC Lomo asks, "If you were an aging professional athlete, presumably over the age of 40, and you didn't have what you used to, and you weren't keeping up with the younger athletes, would you give up, retire, and get soft, or would you work harder to regain what you've lost?" More specifically, if you wanted to improve your game now, even if your joints ached and you were less flexible than before, would you train and work out harder or easier? "Of sure, harder," he says.

You have undoubtedly lost some of your youth's privileges, so you must train harder — and smarter — to compensate for what the years have taken, gradually and unnoticed, as a normal part of the aging process. But, as TC Lomo points out, you didn't have a 40-year expiration date tattooed on your rear when you were born, so what's stopping you from getting back into the muscle-building and fitness game and doing it better than ever before?

The Training Game's New Rules

If training hard and training smart is the formula for success after the age of 40, there are a set of rules, or guidelines, that will get you there faster, easier, and more effectively than picking up a barbell, pulling a cable, stretching a rubber exercise band, or dropping into the plank position and knocking out some push-ups.

The chapters that follow will walk you through the individual activities, but these recommendations are intended to offer you the overall picture, the perspective, on what to do and why to do it.

A brief explanation: Reps are the number of times you lift or pull the weight repeatedly. The repetitions add up to form one set. As an example, an upper-arm workout could consist of three sets of eight reps of barbell curls, with a one-minute break between sets.

1. Take a deep breath. You are probably not near to a high degree of aerobic conditioning unless you have been working hard on the cardiovascular side and have been running, race walking, cycling, swimming, or hitting the elliptical machine or stair climber with adequate frequency and intensity. "I get that, for cardiovascular health and to help keep the pounds off, I need to deal with it, but later, because I want to get started with weightlifting first," you may think. Yes, cardio training has tremendous long-term benefits, but this is about putting you in shape for the short term, to guarantee that you have the aerobic capacity to breathe and function while lifting weights. This aerobic training will take 10 to 20 minutes to begin with and will take place three or four days a week while you complete your resistance workouts. Don't force your heart rate up at first; instead, warm up slowly for two or three minutes. Pick up the pace such that you are breathing hard and deeply for one minute, then slow down for one minute, then pick up the pace again with vigor for one minute, slow, then fast again.

Finish with a one-minute pause.

This is a condensed version of HIIT, or high-intensity interval training, which is a type of aerobic conditioning. It saves time over slower, drawn-out exercise and has been shown to boost the growth and vitality of mitochondria, the energy manufacturers in our muscle cells.

Perform this aerobic activity before, not after, you begin weightlifting. Your goal is to oxygenate your muscle cells before the tension that resistance exercises cause. It is also preferable to gradually warm up your heart muscle rather than driving it up with eight reps of heavy lifting.

2. Put in the effort. You will be working hard whether you like to lift heavy or light weights.

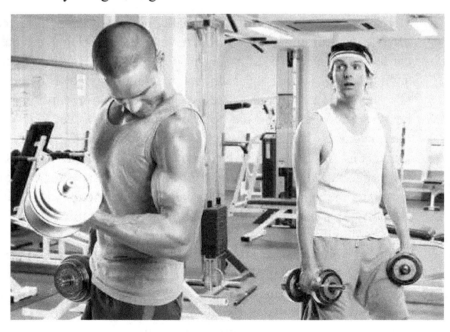

Some professionals believe that lifting higher weights with fewer reps is the greatest method to catch up with where you left off, or where you need to start if this is all new to you. That is not to mean that you will be straining, but many experts advise against doing a lot of reps with light weights. They claim that lifting lesser weights for more reps will help increase endurance but will not help build muscle mass or strength.

Some coaches suggest the opposite approach: lifting lesser weights and performing more reps. For example, instead of lifting a big weight for eight to ten reps, you raise a lesser weight for 15 to 20 reps. Lighter weights have the advantage of putting less strain on joints, tendons, and ligaments, and because every one of us responds differently to physical effort and stress, you must be the final judge of what works best for you. The chapters that follow will go over the numerous workouts and workout programs that you can do.

3. Deal with the discomfort. The phrase "no pain, no gain" became popular in the 1980s when weightlifting and other sports were prominent.

The calisthenics trend began to gain traction. This term was later chastised for pushing people to push themselves beyond their capabilities, which could result in ailments ranging from torn tendons and muscles to joint damage. Today, we know that the responsible way is to push yourself to your boundaries without beyond them. Pain is a signal that should not be ignored.

Lifting large weights can result in a range of aches and pains. Joints can creak and pain and muscles can scream when pushed hard to complete the last rep of a set. These are generally acceptable, but only within certain parameters. Give that last rep your all, but don't overdo it. Give it your all, but don't torture yourself.

Be extra cautious with your shoulders because that group of muscles, known as the rotator cuff, is prone to tears when subjected to shock or severe stress. Most of your skeletal muscles will ache too much for you to injure them, forcing you to back off or halt the activity, but your shoulders give a minimal warning when they are in danger.

4. **Heavy, but not overly** so. Some weightlifters engage in powerlifting, which involves doing very few reps with very high weights. This is not for you since your joints and connective tissues are no longer as flexible and resilient as they were 20 years ago. If you choose to lift heavier weights, make sure the weight isn't too heavy so that you can't accomplish at least eight reps without difficulty. The weight is too heavy if you can only do three or four reps. Reduce the weight until you can perform eight to ten reps at a time.

Keep in mind that growing muscle and strength requires time and patience. Losing the excess weight, you're wanting to lose is also important. That is why, once again, motivation is insufficient; you must commit to going the distance, putting in the months, and then making it a part of your lifestyle for the years ahead.

5. **Rest, but not excessively**. The importance of rest and recuperation time has been hammered home by this point; you got it, muscles.

Get damaged and require time to repair, rebuild, and overbuild

Rest is required for hypertrophy. The ideal quantity for a weightlifter over the age of 40 is 48 hours. Those two days are just what your body requires to rebuild the muscles and get them ready for action. When you were younger, one day of rest would have sufficed, but at this point in your life, that extra day is required. As you discovered earlier in this chapter, rushing to return to the weights can cause more harm than benefit.

However, there is a limit. Too much rest causes the muscles to get lethargic, forget the conditioning, and soften. So, two or three days of recuperation between weightlifting workouts are ideal, four or five days is a little too much, and six or more days is excessive. Never be concerned about missing one scheduled workout day; instead, have the self-discipline to catch up sooner rather than later. Each workout is an investment that you want to protect.

Let's go on to Chapter 3, which discusses how much

You should lift some weight.

CHAPTER 3

How Much Should You Lift?

When it comes to the "how much" question, there are two main camps: how much weight should a middle-aged individual lift? One school of thought holds that you should lift heavier weights with fewer reps per set, while another holds that you should go easy on the weight and give the effort more reps.

Should you, for example, lift a 50-pound barbell eight to ten times to finish one set, or a 2-pound barbell 16 to 20 times every set? What about going to greater extremes, such as using a 9-pound weight for a maximum of two reps or performing 30 to 40 reps with a 12- to 15-pound barbell?

Avoid going to extremes. We can eliminate the extremes for reasons of safety and efficacy. Lifting a weight that you can only lift cleanly and accurately one, two, or three times is not recommended for anyone over the age of 40 whose joints, ligaments, and tendons are no longer as supple and robust as when the person was 20 years younger. Lifting relatively light weights for 30 or more repetitions in a set is also not suggested since, while it is safe and unlikely to cause injury, the effects on growing muscle and strength will be negligible.

There are more reasonable alternatives between the extremes: one that emphasizes muscular hypertrophy and growing strength, and one that delivers the benefits of endurance and muscle toning with less danger of injury or strain.

Heavier Weight Alternatives

The term "heavy" means different things to different individuals and in different contexts. A 10-pound weight is regarded as heavy if held at arm's length, yet light if lifted with a 10-pound barbell. The weight of the weights you lift should be determined by the desired outcome, safety, and degree of exertion.

Somewhat heavyweights

Advocates of the relatively heavier weight technique feel that being a middle-aged weightlifter does not preclude you from lifting heavy weights. If you want to build lean, well-defined muscle mass in the quickest amount of time, moderately heavier weights are the way to go. Advocates' experiences lead them to the belief that the appropriate weight and number of reps per set provide optimal muscle-building benefits while not overtaxing joints and connective tissues.

How heavy is it? It's simple to identify your safe level of considerably bigger weights at any point in your progression cycle because your capacity grows in direct proportion to your strength:

➤ Your capacity is determined by the number of reps you can perform within a given weight range, with eight to ten reps being the ideal number in a set.

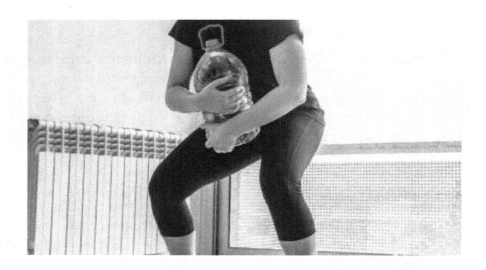

This indicates that you can easily lift the first six or seven reps, but eight, nine, or even ten are challenging. You should be able to reach this level, but not any higher. This calculation must be performed for each weightlifting exercise: arms, shoulders, chest, upper body, core and abdominals, back, and legs, to optimize the training for each muscle group.

If you can only complete five, six, or seven reps, the weight is too heavy; if you can complete more than ten reps, the weight is too light.

You will need to increase the weight level regularly as your strength improves, and when you reach the point where the weight that was difficult to raise fully on the eighth to tenth rep is no longer as difficult, and you can now do more reps. If the weight can be lifted or pulled more than 10 times, the resistance should be increased rather than the reps. Make sure that while you're lifting and counting reps, you're performing the exercises correctly: no jerking or half-lifts.

Weights: Ultra-Heavy vs. Moderately Heavy

You might be curious about powerlifting. Many seasoned, accomplished weightlifters are adamant that the best way to grow muscle mass for both men and women is to lift very heavy weights and gradually raise the weight. Competitive bodybuilders and powerlifters, on the other hand, complete relatively few reps (one to three at most) while lifting extremely large weights that are 90 percent to 100 percent of their maximum in a single rep. Bodybuilding and strength optimization is at least a profound interest for these weightlifters, and for some, it's how they make a job, so they do what works.

Why does this extreme lifting work? Lifting more weight, for example, at least 70% of a person's maximum one-rep weight, stimulates "fast-twitch type 2 muscle fibers, which play an important role in improving muscle strength and stimulating hypertrophy, which is the process of expanding the size of muscle fiber cells."

However, there is a drawback. While type 2 muscle fibers gain more power, they also experience early exhaustion, and muscle fiber stimulation is dependent on how long they are under strain from resistance. If the muscle fibers are not under enough tension for an extended period, they will be less able to commence hypertrophy.

Even more importantly, ultra-heavy weights are not advised for middle-aged weightlifters. A muscle, tendon, or ligament can be pulled or torn with just one rep of extremely large weight.

This signifies that you, at the age of 40 or older, are moderately

Heavy weights are better than ultra-heavy weights:

➢ Because of worries about ultra-heavy lifting, many aspiring weightlifters are finding success with the moderately heavy approach: eight to ten reps at 70 to 75 percent of your maximal one-time lift. (No need to bring anything.)

bringing a calculator to the gym; Determine the weight at which you can do at least eight reps but no more than ten; this is your ideal moderately heavy weight aim.)

The Lighter Weight Alternative

Consider the alternative to lifting greater weights: many reps with weights (or resistance) that you can lift many more times before achieving your maximal effort. We already know that lesser weights are less dangerous since they put less strain on the joints, muscles, tendons, and ligaments. Can smaller weights help you create larger, more defined muscles while also increasing your strength?

Less is More

These are the results of increasing the number of reps in a larger range, such as at least 15 reps per set or even 20 or more. Some people who prefer smaller weights may perform up to 32 reps before calling it a day. The specific weight you can manage when doing numerous reps is considered to be 50-60% of the greatest weight you can lift in a single rep. Determining your ideal lower weight is similar to determining your ideal moderately heavier weight, except now it's determining the highest weight you can lift 20 to 24 times consecutively.

After 24 reps, you may feel as if you have worked hard, and you have! However, the research indicates that you did not lift enough weight to induce a type 2 fast twitch response, which is required to achieve large muscular growth.

Workouts with higher reps and lower weights, on the other hand, have their own set of advantages because they engage different muscle fibers known as type 1, or "slow-twitch muscle fibers." These responses may not generate as much muscle as type 2 responses and produce less power, but they do increase endurance and fatigue slower.

As a result, an exercise with smaller weights and more reps will not necessarily increase your strength but will increase your physical endurance. Higher reps burn more calories since these longer workouts assist burn fat as well as carbohydrates, lowering your total body fat level and giving you a leaner, toned appearance. Your post-workout glow will be stronger, and you will be less likely to endure the agony associated with bigger weights.

To summarise, there are benefits to both lifting lesser weights and performing more reps and lifting relatively heavy weights and doing fewer reps:

When compared to lifting considerably heavier weights and more reps, lesser weights and more reps will not grow muscle or strength.

You will gain muscular endurance and reduce your chance of joint, ligament, tendon, or muscle damage by lifting weights.

Lifting fairly heavy weights will help you achieve your muscle-building and strength-building goals, but be aware that there is a greater danger of strain or injury. Take care not to overdo the weights, and let the number of reps guide you. It's too heavy if you can't raise it eight times.

Celebrity Weightlifters in their Forties

Becoming a weightlifter after the age of 40, or returning to weightlifting after a long break, is nothing new or unusual. Men and women who do not want to accept the bad effects of adulthood and who want to halt the aging process and retain good health, on the other hand, are working out with weights at health clubs, fitness centers, gyms, and at home.

Their routines may differ from person to person, but they share the similar goal of wanting to get stronger and look stronger.

Middle-aged people working out, increasing their musculature, getting stronger, and shaping up is all around us, and a visit to a fitness center will confirm that it's not just younger people who are curling dumbbells, lifting barbells, swinging kettle weights, pulling cables, stretching exercise bands, and doing pull-ups. Treadmills, ellipticals, and cycles are often used by elderly men and women who incorporate a good cardiovascular workout into their daily routines.

Other examples of middle-aged weightlifting and physical fitness supporters include action-hero superstars such as Jason Statham, Daniel Craig, Dwayne "The Rock" Johnson, and Hugh Jackman.

Statham, Jason

The Mechanic, Furious 7, Death Race, and Hobbs & Shaw are just a few of Jason Statham's flicks. We know him as an action hero scaling skyscrapers, overcoming foes, and being an all-around tough guy in these and many other films and shows. But Jason is no child, and at 52, he's working out as hard as he's ever worked out, reminiscent of his days as a diver and footballer. That is why he has an outstanding physique and seems and feels like his younger self.

What is his daily routine? Jason's goals are to maintain lean muscle, lose excess body fat, and remain strong and flexible. He wants to keep his metabolism going, and he attributes his fitness to both his food and his workouts.

We'll go through his diet in more detail later, but here are the highlights of what he consumes.

A sensible diet. Jason appears to follow a Mediterranean-style diet that includes oats and other healthy grains, nuts and seeds, cold-water fish (rich in omega-3 antioxidants), lean poultry, brown rice, plenty of fresh fruit, and a variety of vegetables. Protein is essential for muscular growth. He estimates that around 95 percent of his diet is healthy, though he does allow himself some chocolate (dark chocolate is now acknowledged as good, so there is no reason for guilt). To his credit and nutritional benefit, he avoids fatty fried foods (as should everyone worried about their health).

A full day of Jason's nutritional choices will be shown in Chapter 6, but here are some highlights to give you a sense of what makes a good diet for a middle-aged athlete who wants to get stronger, stay fit, and stay healthy:

Breakfast starts with fresh fruits like strawberries and pineapple, then oatmeal with cholesterol-lowering fiber, and finally poached eggs for a protein boost.

Brown rice, which contains great carbohydrates, fiber, vitamins, minerals, and some protein, is frequently served for lunch. Jason includes steamed veggies for extra nutrients; this combo is a vegan meal that he enjoys on occasion. He frequently adds a bowl of hot miso soup, which Jason thinks is wonderful and healthful (it is, but be cautious of the salt level if you have high blood pressure).

Snack time is not the time since he enjoys crunching on cashews, almonds, and walnuts. Peanut butter contains nuts, but not processed, sugar-laden commercial kinds. Jason prefers the unprocessed, all-natural variety, which is made entirely of ground peanuts.

(Again, salt is bad for you; salt-free is healthier.)

Dinner is the higher protein meal, with lean beef one night and chicken or fish the next. Salmon or other cold-water fish are the best options and chicken should be lean.

Jason's evening meal consists of veggies as well as a leafy green salad. (Hint: If you start your evening meal with a huge green salad, you'll eat fewer of the higher-calorie dishes that follow.)

A fantastic exercise. Here's one day of Jason's seven-day fitness regimen. This is his workout, not yours, so be motivated to do it someday. More practically, tell yourself that if he can do all that powerlifting, what you'll learn in the next chapter will be a piece of cake.

Remember, Jason Statham has been working out with increasing intensity his entire life, so don't feel like you're falling short. If Jason were starting an exercise program in his forties or returning to weightlifting after a 15- or 20-year sabbatical, he'd probably be following the same plan you'll be doing.

His actual Day 1 is as follows:

Progression of One-Rep Max Deadlifts

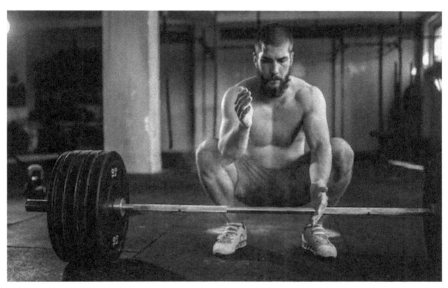

A series of warm-ups and one-rep bench press workouts prepare you for a single goal: the almighty deadlift (a one-repetition max of the largest weight you can lift at one time).

Jason begins by rowing for 10 minutes at a moderate tempo as a warm-up to get the blood flowing and the muscles oxygenated. Then, using a lightweight and his bodyweight, he performs one rep of each of the following three exercises: barbell squat, press-up (same as push-up), and ring pull-ups. One round of the circuit is completed, then repeated with two reps; stop, then repeat for three reps, four reps, and five reps. Then he lowers the circuit with four reps, three reps, two reps, and one rep.

Jason is now warmed up and ready to go to work. If simply reading about his warm-up makes you tired, buckle up for what's about to come.

The ultra-heavy weightlifting we covered in the last part, Jason Statham's deadlift program, is not for you. But Jason has a plan, and it's right here.

The one-rep maximum weight routine is known as a deadlift. You can see that he starts heavy, then gets heavier, and finally reaches 365 pounds. Jason's deadlift routine for the barbell squat is as follows:

1. 10 reps of 135-pound lifting, followed by a one-minute break.

2. 5 reps of 185-pound lifting, followed by a two-minute break.

3. 3 reps of 235-pound lifting, followed by a three-minute break.

4. 2 reps of 285-pound lifting, followed by a three-minute break.

5. One rep of 325 pounds followed by a three-minute break.

6. 6. 1 rep of 350 pounds lifted, followed by a three-minute break.

7. 1 rep of 360-pound lifting, followed by a three-minute break.

8. Lift 365 pounds for one rep, then rest for three minutes before cooling down.

Relax for a while. Jason is practicing footwork for 10 minutes on a trampoline; an option is maybe 10 to 15 minutes on a treadmill at a modest pace and elevation.

While the amount of weight lifted is astounding, take note of how the weights are gradually increased and how the rest between lifts rises as the weights climb. Yes, the ultimate weight is quite heavy, but Jason progressively built up to it with proper rest between lifts.

Day 2 consists of five separate exercises, all done in sequence, that is less about weights and more about reps. Jason refers to this as the Big Five 55 Workout. He alternates between five exercises: front squats, pull-ups, push-ups, power clean lifts (bend down, lift the barbell to the chest, hold erect, then descend), and dragging knees up to elbows while hanging on the pull-up bar.

He performs 10 sets with minimal rest in between, totaling 55 reps for each of the five exercises.

Statham cycles between the five exercises, completing the circuit ten times. He starts with ten reps, then nine, then eight, and so on, for a total of 55 reps per exercise. Each set should be followed by a short period of rest.

For a change of pace, Day 3 is fully aerobic and done entirely on the rowing machine. He warms up gently on the machine for 10 minutes before performing six high-intensity sprints, each covering 500 meters in one minute and 40 seconds, which is extremely quick. He cools off by walking 500 meters with two big kettle weights on his back.

Craig, Daniel

Daniel Craig, the most robust and powerful of the James Bond actors, appears to be capable of dealing with any situation or foe. His training has resulted in a physique that appears powerful, yet functional, with flexibility, speed, and significant strength. How does he work out?

He begins the week with a power circuit that works the entire body, not just one or two muscle groups, and consists of three sets of ten reps. This series comprises workouts for the arms and shoulders, chest, abdominals and core, upper and lower back, and legs, which include glutes, quadriceps, hamstrings, and calves. Daniel will exercise only a few muscle groups for the following four days, performing four sets of ten reps. Every session ends with a five-minute sprint interval on the treadmill or outside the gym. His trainer then instructs him to skip the gym over the weekend, but to perform some mild yoga-style stretching and easy aerobic workouts, such as a slow to moderate-paced swim or run.

Workout on Day 2. Daniel's Day 2 muscle group, for example, works the chest, shoulders, and back.

The program comprises four movements that you can try because they involve relatively heavy weights and are performed for 10 reps each:

1. Bench press using an inclined barbell. The beginning position is reclining back on an incline bench. With the palms facing forward, the barbell is hoisted to shoulder height. Exhale completely and raise the barbell with both arms. Hold in the fully extended posture for a few seconds, then inhale and slowly return to the beginning position. Daniel does four sets of ten reps, with 90-second breaks in between.

2. Pull-ups are a calisthenic workout that begins with reaching up to hold the pull-up bar or handles with palms facing front and hands about shoulder-width apart. Slowly raise your chin to the level of the bar.

or handles, then gradually lower to the starting position.

Lift and exhale while squeezing your shoulder blades.

Inhale as you lower yourself back down. Perform four sets of ten reps, with 90-second breaks in between.

3. Incline press-ups are a modified version of the basic push-up that are slightly easier to perform because you are not lowering down and pulling up from the floor position. Put your hands shoulder-width apart on a bench and completely extend your legs to the back. You need to be on your toes. Starting with your arms fully extended, carefully lower your chest to the bench, inhaling as you go.

Pause for a time, then fully return to the beginning posture, breathing as you do so. Perform four sets of ten reps, resting 90 seconds between sets.

4. Begin the dumbbell incline fly by lying on an incline bench with a dumbbell in each hand. Start with your arms completely extended upward. Lower your arms out to the side slowly until they are parallel to the floor, or as far as you can comfortably lower them without pain. A small bend at the elbow may be more comfortable. Repeat the technique by raising your arms above your head again.

Perform four sets of ten reps with 90-second rests between sets, the same as the other exercises in this group.

On other days, Daniel Craig does leg strengthening workouts as well as bicep curls and dips for his arms and shoulders.

shoulders. Then comes the weekend with no weights, followed by a full-body workout on Monday after a two-day break.

"The Rock" Dwayne Johnson

The Rock is well-known for his transition from college athlete to WWE phenom to action movie hero. Unlike many other well-built Hollywood stars, Dwayne may be the best-built, most muscular star of all time, with the possible exception of Arnold Schwarzenegger. Dwayne makes it clear that he worked hard to reach where he is and to attain his massive muscles, but he is always willing to share his knowledge and methods with others. While few of us aspire to the muscle size he displayed in Fast Five or Hercules, or to be anywhere near Dwayne's level, there may be a benefit in allowing him to impart his advice. He is, without a doubt, inspirational.

He begins with cardio. Every morning, The Rock goes to the elliptical cross-training machine for 30 to 50 minutes of vigorous aerobics.

Then there's breakfast. He starts his day by filling it up with a protein-rich breakfast. For example, on most days, he has five substantial meals, the first of which, following early cardio and a shower, involves no less than:

2 cups cooked oatmeal (start with 1 cup dried oats)

3 egg whites plus 1 full egg (egg whites are nearly 100% protein)

10 oz. steak or some lean meat (for extra protein)

1 glass of watermelon juice

The remaining four or five meals of the day include an eight-ounce amount of fish, poultry, or beef, as well as vegetables such as broccoli, asparagus, and potato, as well as plenty of eggs and egg whites. The final meal consists of 10 egg whites and casein protein.

Later in the morning, the workout begins. The Rock makes things as difficult and intense as he can to adhere to his philosophy of "epic pain, epic gain." This is not a fitness regimen that you should try to mimic, but what Dwayne does

His journey to obtain his huge muscles and the razor-sharp definition demonstrates what the human body is capable of.

Even a small portion of these muscles can be amazing.

He works out six days a week and changes his routine from day to day to rest different muscle groups and keep things interesting.

The legs are the emphasis of Day 1.

Take note of the moderate to high rep range.

The second day is dedicated to the back and shoulder muscles.

Squat with a barbell: 4 sets of 12 reps

4 sets of 12 reps on the thigh abductor

4 sets of 12 repetitions of hack squat

4 sets of 25 reps on the leg press

Leg extensions: three sets of twenty reps

4 sets of 12 repetitions of single-leg hack squat

4 sets of 10 repetitions on the Romanian Deadlift

Walking Lunge with a Barbell: 4 sets of 25 reps

3 sets of 20 reps of seated leg curls

3 sets of pull-ups to failure

4 sets of 12 reps on the bent-over barbell row

Lat Pulldown 4 sets of 12 repetitions on the pulldown

Barbell Bending 4 sets of 12 repetitions on the row

4 sets of 12 reps of one-arm dumbbell row

Barbell 3 sets of 10 repetitions on the deadlift

3 sets of inverted rowing to failure

4 sets of 12 repetitions of dumbbell shrug

4 sets of 12 reps of back hyperextensions

The week continues on Day 3 with shoulders, Day 4 with arms and abs, Day 5 with legs again, and Day 6 with the chest. Day 7 is a leisure day with no workouts, and The Rock is said to eat ice cream on this day once a week. It appears to be well merited.

Hugh Jackman's bio

Hugh Jackman bulked up well-defined muscles in the 17 years he played Wolverine, a mutant with steel knife-blade hands, in the X-Men movies by following a demanding gym routine and a high-protein diet. His career has progressed from action hero to leading man in the musical Les Misérables.

A well-balanced diet. Hugh's diet has always included extra protein, but he is not a protein-obsessed maniac. He supplements his diet with healthy, unprocessed carbs such as sweet potatoes, broccoli, spinach, and avocado.

It contains omega-3 antioxidants as well as niacin, beta-carotene, riboflavin, folate, magnesium, potassium, and pantothenic acid

as well as vitamins Whole grains, particularly oatmeal and brown rice, provide carbs and protein while also being strong in antioxidants, vitamins, minerals, and digestion-friendly fiber. Oats are also thought to reduce LDL (bad) cholesterol.

Eggs, fish for omega-3 fats, poultry, and lean beef are all good sources of protein. Overall, it's a protein-rich version of the Mediterranean diet; however, there's no indication that he also eats nuts, seeds, and beans.

Muscle gain and muscle loss Hugh's trainer introduced him to a dual strategy workout routine, one of which focused on muscle building.

One aims to increase muscle mass, while the other aims to create a better definition. To emphasize leanness, low-intensity/high-intensity intervals were included.

muscle and reduce body fat

Hugh's training has been based on progressive overload, which involves gradually increasing the weight being pulled, pushed, and lifted during each workout to ensure consistent strength gains.

The weight was increased for the first three weeks of a four-week cycle, then decreased for the fourth week with a corresponding increase in the number of reps.

According to this four-week regimen with progressions throughout the first three weeks, Hugh performed the following exercises: barbell bench press, back squat, weighted pullup, and barbell deadlift.

Hugh Jackman's four-week progressive overload plan:

Set one: 5 repetitions at 60% of max, set two: 5 reps at 65% of max

Set three consists of 5 repetitions at 70% of the maximum.

Set four consists of 5 repetitions at 75% of the maximum.

Week 2:

4 repetitions at 65% of max in set one; 4 reps at 75% max in set two

Set three consists of four reps at 85% of one's maximum.

Set four consists of four reps at 85% of one's maximum.

Week 3:

3 repetitions at 70% of max in set one; 3 reps at 80% max in set two

Set three consists of three reps at 90% of one's maximum.

Set four consists of three reps at 90% of one's maximum.

Week 4:

Set one: 10 reps at 40% of max; set two: 10 reps at 50% of max.

Set three consists of 10 repetitions at 60% of the maximum.

Set four consists of 10 reps at 90% of one's maximum.

Surprisingly, Hugh's trainer limited his training to only five major exercises to strengthen his arms and shoulders, chest, abs, back, and legs.

Now that you're motivated to gain muscles and start a successful weightlifting and fitness program, it's time to move on to Chapter 4's action plan.

CHAPTER 4

Exercise Routines and Recovery Techniques

With the lessons and insights, we've already covered, and an understanding of why heavier weights have an advantage over lighter weights, you're now ready to design your training and recuperation plan. This chapter will teach you about the many exercise routines that you can use to create a unique, successful fitness regimen. While you will be performing many of your exercises with big weights, they may not be as heavy as the weights you lifted when you were younger (if you ever lifted weights at all) or that you see others lifting.

Weightlifting isn't only about iron weights and cable machines. It also contains bodyweight calisthenics, which are routines that use only your body weight to provide the necessary resistance for demanding workouts that yield spectacular results.

Those working out at home without equipment can enhance calisthenics by purchasing stretch bands or tubes that can be used to duplicate many of the routines performed at fitness centers with weights and progressive resistance devices. Weightlifting with weights and bodyweight calisthenics will be covered in this chapter.

Most weightlifting exercises can be performed safely after the age of 40, as long as you work gradually and don't try to lift too much. Maintain complete awareness of the recovery period required after weightlifting to allow hypertrophy, the rebuilding, and the development process, to function, and be aware that after the age of 40, hypertrophy takes longer and the danger of injury from overwork increases. As stated in the opening, patience will be rewarded with results; building lean, well-defined muscles takes time and effort.

The Appropriate Routine for Your Age

Like most number designations, your age is relative. Your capacity to do a variety of weightlifting exercises with varied weights and reps at age 40, 50, or 60 is determined by your current physical condition.

Your condition is determined by several factors, including how aging has affected you, such as the degrees of joint and tendon flexibility and how they may have stiffened; your overall health; whether your muscles have atrophied due to lack of use; and whether your cardiovascular system is fully functional. "It's not the years, it's the miles," as the saying goes, implying that your ailment is caused by damage caused by under or over-use. It is critical to treat your body with respect for its current state rather than what you want or wish it to be. If you want to attain your goals of increased strength, bigger muscles, and general fitness, you must be realistic.

First and foremost, not harm.

Yes, you will work hard and put your muscles, joints, tendons, and ligaments to the test, but your goal is to strengthen and expand, not punish and harm.

Whatever your current state, respect your body as a middle-aged one and adhere to the Hippocratic principle of "first, not harm." Even if you start with the finest of intentions, exercising in ways that are best left to seasoned, well-conditioned athletes, or attempting to lift more weight than your joints can handle

You are putting your ligaments at undue risk:

The injury might range from a torn rotator cuff in your shoulder to a strained muscle that holds your kneecap in place. This type of injury might take months to recover. Working within your skill level poses little risk of injury.

Overuse means that the muscles have been overextended, and the damage done to the fibers and cells will not be repaired or recovered within the standard two days of rest. As a result, muscles do not expand and may atrophy, or shrink.

Pain, because lifting or pulling too much weight or performing too many reps can hurt and reduce your excitement and motivation for strength training. Consider pain to be a warning sign.

You are unique because of your age, physical condition, health, and other aspects. This is why you are advised not to pay attention to other weightlifters. They have limitations, and you have yours. Over lifting, pushing, or pulling too much too early in your middle age return to weightlifting, only to harm yourself with a strained or torn muscle and shut down what you have just started, has no value.

Middle-Age Exercises to Avoid

Aside from lifting too much weight, there are several popular workouts that you may be familiar with and intend to incorporate into your regimen, but specialists urge you to abandon them to prevent the danger of injury. Tell yourself that you've outgrown these exercises and pass them on to the kids:

The overhead press. Standing with a barbell above your head and lowering it to your shoulders behind your head places undue strain on your shoulders, neck, and spine.

Bench pressing Lying on a bench and lifting a heavy barbell upwards may be beneficial for your chest when you're 25, but by 45, you're putting too much strain on your pectoral (chest) muscles, wrists, and shoulders.

Crunches. These modest lifts of the head and shoulders while lying on your back replaced the sit-up as a safer alternative, but crunches put too much pressure on your neck and spine in middle age. By performing leg rises, hanging leg raises, and planks, you may avoid pinched nerves and work your abs with less danger.

Deadlifts. Bending over and lifting a barbell to your chest is bad for your back. Deadlifts, at the very least, can create chronic back pain and may result in more serious back injuries.

Leg pressure Sitting and moving a large weight with your legs bent may appear to be harmless, but the pressure on middle-aged hips and knees can cause joint pain. Instead, strengthen your legs with low-impact lunges while holding a light dumbbell or no weight at all.

Pull-downs on the side. You sit on a bench in front of the machine, reach up, and pull a bar to your chest, or worse, behind your neck. This procedure poses a danger of pinched neck nerves and damaged rotator-cuff shoulder muscles in middle age.

While it is suggested to incorporate cardiovascular exercise into your routines, be mindful that running on hard surfaces can cause lifelong knee damage, and you should limit your outdoor running to a treadmill or on grass. Runners should use quality shoes that provide softer landings and assist reduce pronation, or outward foot rotation.

You, Will, Require the Following Equipment (and Alternatives)

Fitness facilities. Strength training involves kinds of resistance that are the foundation of creating lean, defined muscle and being stronger. A health club or fitness center would typically have a full range of weightlifting equipment, such as free weights like dumbbells, barbells, and kettlebells, as well as progressive exercise machines with cables and weights that you may pull or push to work different muscle areas. Rubber stretches tubes, adjustable seats, and a pull-up bar are additional common features in a well-equipped fitness center or gym.

Unless you live in an apartment building or residential neighborhood that includes a fitness facility as a benefit, these fitness clubs normally need monthly membership fees.

The home gym. A smart alternative to a health club membership is to set up your tiny home gym with free weights, a portable pull-up and chin-up bar, and a variety of elastic rubber bands or tubes. The little investment in this equipment may be soon repaid by the savings in monthly fitness facility membership expenses.

Bodyweight exercises. Using your weight as resistance is an even less expensive technique to gain muscle and strength. Push-ups, pull-ups, and chin-ups, as well as leg, raise, planks, and dips, are all examples. Numerous other calisthenics movements can be used to complete a full-body workout.

Weightlifting activities in Group 1 are predicated on having access to weights and other resistance equipment. Group 2 calisthenics is almost entirely equipment-free and can be done at home. You are urged to try exercises from both categories to add diversity to your workouts and provide your muscles with a wider range of demands.

Each exercise includes photos of the movement as well as a link to a YouTube video example to ensure that you learn the motions correctly.

Skip the advertisement. Many of the videos will start with a brief commercial, but after five seconds, a "Skip Ad" box will appear in the lower right corner of the screen, and a single click will launch the exercise demo.

Weightlifting Exercises (Group 1)

The weightlifting routines listed below have been chosen to produce good strength and muscle growth results while posing a low risk of injury. Choose exercises that target certain muscle groups and then vary them so that you have at least one, preferably two, days off before training the same muscle groups again.

Breathe out as you raise and in as you lower the weights.

Tip: Choose a weight that you can lift eight to ten reps with, and execute three sets with 60 to 90 seconds of rest between sets.

1. Incline Dumbbell Press

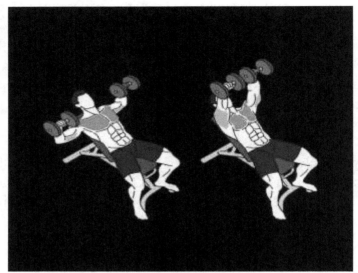

The dumbbell incline press works your chest, upper arms, shoulders, and lats (sides of the upper chest).

When performing the dumbbell incline press for the first few times, use a lesser weight than you believe is suitable.

You don't want to over-lift or struggle to keep the dumbbells under control because they're too heavy.

If the dumbbells are still difficult to handle, try the exercise using a barbell. To imitate the movement with barbells, use a broad grasp (just past shoulder width).

2. Cable Rows While Seated

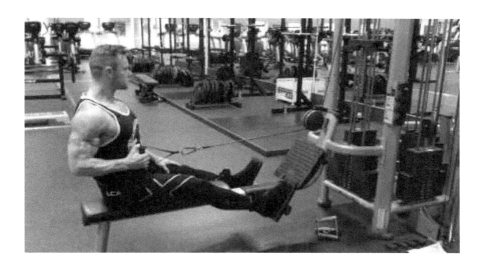

This is a complex workout that strengthens the shoulders.

Abdominals and core muscles, both front and rear

Tip: This is a great workout for the hard-to-reach back muscles, but make sure you draw a weight that you can carry without straining your back.

Squeeze your shoulder blades together as you reach the full extent of the pull-back for extra conditioning.

3. Split Squats with Dumbbells

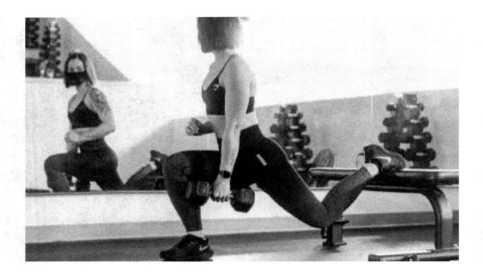

This leg exercise targets the quadriceps and hamstrings.

important muscles on the front of your thighs

Tip: Do not lean backward to keep your equilibrium.

control of the movement is required, but a minor forward tilt is acceptable.

Tip: Perform eight to ten repetitions with the same leg ahead, then transfer to the opposite leg and repeat to complete one set, keeping your weight on the lead foot.

If doing eight reps with each leg is too difficult, use lighter weights and fewer reps the first week; do three sets with a 90-second rest between sets.

"Dumbbell Split Squat - "

4. Dumbbell Bent-Over Rows

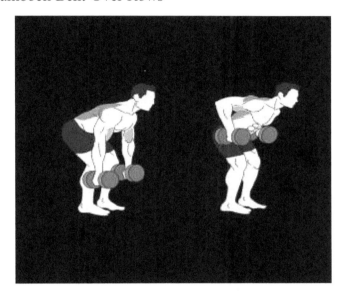

This will isolate your back muscles, particularly the rhomboids, lats, and trapezoids. You will also assist in stabilizing your core and lower body by training the upper arm biceps and posterior deltoids.

If you feel your back hurting, minimize the amount of forwarding bend to relieve pressure on your spine.

Another grip option is to hold the dumbbells with your hands facing back. (You can boost the muscles involved by alternating hold with palms to sides and palms to back between reps or sets.)

"How to: Dumbbell Bend-Over" video demonstration

row,"

5. Upright Dumbbell Row

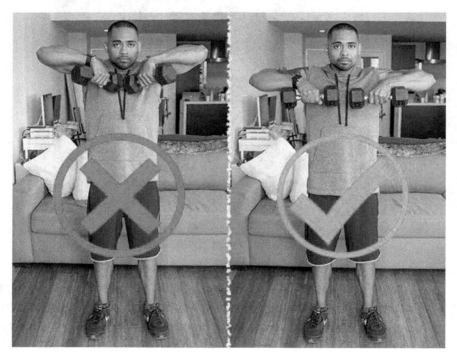

When done correctly, this is an excellent shoulder-strengthening exercise with significant advantages. Trainers warn, however, that if done poorly, upright rows can cause more harm than benefit, so pay special attention to your form. To begin, start with lesser weights to be on the safe side.

Tip: Because you'll be starting with smaller weights for safety, do 12 to 14 reps for each of three sets, with 60 seconds break in between. Reduce the weight you're lifting if you can't do 12 reps.

"How to Properly Row an Upright Row" video demonstration

shape and advice."

Standing Barbell Curl 6

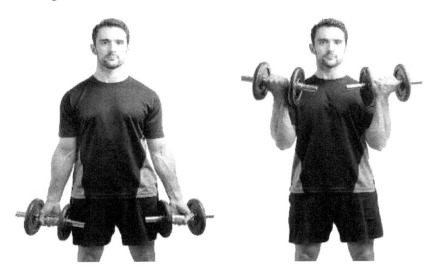

Weightlifters use this workout to build their upper arms, particularly their biceps. It can also be done with two dumbbells, but a barbell is preferable for beginners because it is easier to handle and tends to follow the ideal route of up-and-down movements.

Tip: Lift the bar with both arms exerting equal work (this will keep the bar parallel to the floor), and do not jerk the weight upwards or let it drop down too quickly. Slower is better in weightlifting, as it is in all sports.

Perform three sets of eight to ten reps, resting 60 to 90 seconds between sets if possible. If accomplishing eight reps is too difficult for you, use a lighter barbell.

Consult Your Doctor (2)

Workouts may cause you to visit your doctor for a variety of reasons, including heart-related issues or joint, muscle, or tendon damage. Follow the warning label on most aerobic exercise machines: if you get chest pain, lightheadedness, dizziness, or nausea, stop and seek medical attention. It could be nothing, such as indigestion, or it could be a warning sign that something in your cardiovascular system needs immediate care.

When pain and stiffness in a joint are persistent and interfere with regular activities, it is necessary to consult an orthopedist, many of whom have training in sports medicine and are familiar with exercise-induced injuries. In many circumstances, you will be instructed to use the R.I.C.E. method (rest, ice, compression, and elevation). A cortisone injection may be required to reduce inflammation and aid healing in some joint injuries.

In conclusion, some pain and discomfort are common side effects of lifting weights and exercising out. Use common sense when it comes to the amount of weight you lift, and make sure to follow the rest and recovery protocols. Be aware of when the pain becomes severe, and do not disregard its warnings. The sooner physical disorders are identified and treated, the quicker the recovery.

Now it's on to Chapter 5 for some additional ideas on how to get started.

get your workouts started and keep them continuing

CHAPTER 5

Metabolism, Motivation, and Dedication

The goal of this chapter is to assist you in understanding what will make the difference in your ability to attain the goals you have set for yourself as an aspiring weightlifter and fitness enthusiast. You may have tried weightlifting and bodybuilding in the past but gave up when other commitments demanded your time and attention. Your energy level began to dwindle, and the weights began to become heavier rather than lighter. You may have been a runner once, but it has faded as well.

Or perhaps this is all new to you. You rarely (if ever) lifted weights or did significant bodyweight calisthenics.

Cardiovascular training? Have no time or interest?

Whatever the case may be, you've arrived and are ready to face the challenges and rewards of building more lean muscle, being stronger, and being in overall good, healthy shape. Understandably, you're eager to get started on the weightlifting and bodyweight calisthenics discussed in the last chapter.

But first, take some time to grasp why things are different for you now that you're in your forties.

Continuity in your workouts and attention to your food are crucial for reasons other than working out hard, getting enough rest, and experiencing great outcomes. Things slow down as you become older, and your muscle mass decreases. Why?

The Unseen Factor in Metabolism

Do you ever wonder why a middle-aged person like yourself can't create muscle tissue and gain mass like someone younger?

in his twenties? Why do people in their 40s lose muscle mass faster than people in their 20s? Why does fat seem to accumulate more quickly, and why do the pounds pile on even if you eat the same amount as when you were younger? You must grasp and control an invisible aspect now that you are 40, 50, or older. It is your metabolism, which is the sum of your body's biological and chemical cellular processing. It's slower than it used to be at your age, and your fitness and dietary regimens must be altered to reverse the reduction of your current metabolic rate.

Muscle Mass Loss

Your metabolism slows as a result of lifestyle variables. You may be aware that the majority of middle-aged adults lead a less active, more sedentary lifestyle, which adds to muscle loss, making your dedication to a serious physical fitness plan all the more crucial. Aside from your behavior, it is natural for you to undergo muscle loss and metabolic system aging.

Sarcopenia is the term for age-related muscle loss, which is a normal and natural part of aging. According to Harvard Health Publishing (2016), after the age of 30, you can lose between 3% and 5% of your muscle mass per decade. Men lose more muscle than women; on average, men lose 30% of their muscular mass over their lifetimes.

However, the muscular loss is not unavoidable, and muscle mass can be enhanced rather than diminished by committing to a good weightlifting program of resistance workouts that lasts into middle life.

According to Dr. Thomas W. Storer, director of the physical function and exercise physiology laboratory at Brigham and Women's Hospital, lost muscle mass can be restored. He claims that it requires effort, planning, and attention, but that "it is never too late to rebuild and retain muscle" (2016).

Sarcopenia, or muscle loss, is linked to testosterone reductions, and studies have been done to see if testosterone supplements might slow or reverse muscle mass loss.

While some outcomes were encouraging, there were some negative side effects, and the FDA has not approved testosterone supplements for muscle mass gain in men.

As a result, Dr. Storer finds that, regardless of age, the best way to grow lean muscle mass is a consistent regimen of progressive resistance training:

progressively increasing the amount of time, you spend working out

As your strength and endurance develop, increase the amount of weight lifted while maintaining the number of reps and sets.

Rates of Metabolic Consumption

The number of calories you burn in a day is directly related to your metabolic rate. This calorie consumption rate can be stated in numerous ways:

When you are asleep, immobile, or resting, your resting metabolic rate is assessed. It is the lowest rate that can sustain basic reflexes that keep you alive, such as energy consumption to maintain your heartbeat, breathing, and brain functioning. When you are at rest, you burn the fewest calories each hour.

The caloric consumption required to support digestion of the food you eat and process in a given period, including chewing and swallowing, grinding and acidification in the stomach, and assimilation of food in the small and large intestines as it is carried through the GI tract by peristalsis contractions, is referred to as the thermic effect of food.

Non-exercise thermogenesis refers to all calories burned while standing, sitting, writing, reading, speaking, laughing, doing light housework, and doing anything else that requires physical effort other than exercise and digesting.

The number of calories burned during and soon after exercise is referred to as exercise consumption. Walking, gardening, lifting and carrying, showering, stair climbing, jogging and running quickly, weightlifting, swimming, and cycling are all examples of active exercise.

The number of calories expended by these four categories varies depending on individual metabolic rates and other factors such as the type, amount, and intensity of the workouts and motions performed. Your \metabolic rate can be altered by your age and certain physical

Muscle mass, height, weight, genetics, and hormones are all factors to consider.

We'll talk about calories and weight loss in the following chapter, but it's crucial to remember that weight increase, weight maintenance, and weight loss are all influenced by two factors: the number of calories taken and assimilated, and the number of calories metabolized.

Any calories consumed more than your daily requirements that are not expended are stored as fat.

Increase Your Metabolism

Let's have a look at your metabolic control alternatives. Can you impact the rate at which your metabolism burns calories, especially because your metabolic rate slows with age?

Exercise and other physical activity can boost your metabolism immediately and have a secondary effect during rest and even sleep:

Non-exercise thermogenesis can be influenced by becoming less sedentary and more active during the day.

Avoid sitting while working by placing your laptop or desktop computer keyboard at a height that allows you to work in a standing position at least part of the time. Take the stairs instead of the elevator, do your chores, and integrate some yoga stretching into your day (or Tai chi or Pilates). Being more active and less sedentary daily can help you burn an extra 200, 600, or more calories while also keeping you more flexible and healthier overall.

Exercise thermogenesis can be a more efficient technique to burn calories. The volume and intensity of the exercises are closely proportional to the calories burned; thus a 40-minute weightlifting session can burn 500 to 600 calories compared to 40 to 80 calories ingested during the same period sitting and watching TV or conversing. Similarly, two miles of running or brisk walking on the treadmill can burn 200 to 220 calories in 20 to 30 minutes, compared to 20 or so calories eaten when sitting.

Muscle growth: According to research, the age-related metabolic slowdown is linked to muscle mass loss, thus using weightlifting to develop muscle mass will result in a higher total metabolism rate even during the sleeping and resting phases, when the metabolic rate is at its slowest. A 10% rise in resting metabolic rate can result in hundreds of additional calories burned overnight with little effort on your side!

The most effective discipline combines both of these practices: being more active and less sedentary throughout the day, which can raise your metabolism; and exercising with weightlifting and aerobics at least three days each week. You can't change your metabolism by changing how your body digests and absorbs nutrients, but adding extra physical activity to your daily routine can increase your calorie burn rate even when you're resting or sleeping.

Appetite effects: Here's a heads-up to warn you of a weight-related impact that may surprise you. Despite a weightlifting and aerobics regimen, it can cause you to gain weight rather than lose or maintain your present weight:

Increased exercise and daily activity will burn more calories, but it will also likely boost your appetite. This can result in consuming more calories than you burn.

Avoid snacking excessively, and when you do, prioritize lean protein, which will keep you feeling fuller for longer (protein is slower to digest) and is advantageous to the muscle-building process of hypertrophy.

Motivation and dedication

Mental power is a vital component of your long-term muscle and strength-building regimen. Of course, the weights will be included.

The reps, sets, and pauses in between will give you the lean muscle mass you need, but your mental state will determine whether you start and if you will stick with it for the months and years of training required. Rome was not built in a day, and your outstanding figure will not appear overnight.

The Inspiration

The necessity of motivation was presented in the first chapter and at different places throughout this book as an incentive to get your weightlifting and fitness program started. No one can force you to start a regular, well-planned weightlifting program; you must have the determination and desire to take care of your body, health, and appearance:

If you've made it this far, you're probably aware that "you're in."

You visualize yourself lifting barbells and dumbbells, performing push-ups and pull-ups, planks, squats, and splits.

You are committed to cardiovascular conditioning to help you lose weight while investing in your health and longevity.

You feel better gazing in the mirror, anticipating the larger, more defined muscles you will develop.

The Engagement

But will you have the will and discipline to go the distance, to continue with your bodybuilding and strengthening workouts daily? Motivation is vital at first, but you must have the discipline to stay in the program even on days when you don't feel like it, when you say, "I'll do it tomorrow."

You need to transcend the forces that hold you back, to \ break free of the restraints, and be devoted no matter how \stirred or uninspired you are at that moment. Only then will you be able to stay on track to reach your fitness and strength goals.

Commitment to success as a weightlifter, who develops muscle, and loses fat, and extra weight, begins in the mind, which is the most effective and convincing instrument that will assist you in achieving your bodybuilding goals. A positive attitude and the determination to work through the most difficult movements will get you through the roughest times with tenacity. Those who fail, give up, or quit may be physically tough, but they lack mental toughness. Keep in mind that your body will always follow your intellect.

Successful weightlifters at all levels of training have developed positive thinking to arrive at the gym, take up the first weight of the session, and complete it with a full effort, regardless of how fatigued or busy they were. You may adopt these concepts, make them yours, and allow them to carry you to the gym and through the day's job every time.

Positive Discipline

1. I'll do a half-workout today and relax.

This is useful when you're fatigued and helps you get started. In virtually every situation, after you get started and warmed up, you get into the exercises, complete all of the reps, and complete the entire workout. It's a little psychological game you can play on yourself that strangely works time after again. As the saying goes, "simply showing up is 90% of success," so put on your training shoes and shorts, choose a machine or a weight, and begin cautiously. You'll get toasty and keep going.

2. The focus and discipline of a single mountain climber.

There is no gazing up or down when ascending the edge of Yosemite's El Capitan without ropes or gear. There is no thinking about what's ahead or how difficult it will be. The same is true for weightlifting when all that matters is what you need to do right now: focus on the now. Another advantage of working out in the present moment is that it allows you to clear your thoughts in a meditative manner, allowing you to disregard any distractions. You will be calmer, and by paying close attention, your form and posture will improve, making you less likely to injure yourself.

3. A mirror, a scale, and a tape measure

The figures do not lie, exaggerate, or try to appease your ego. They are the facts that will bear witness to the depth and duration of your dedication to building your body, losing weight, and flattening your stomach. Begin with a baseline set of measures and check in every week. Look in the mirror without judgment or disappointment and just note how your pecs (chest muscles) and abdominals look: a touch soft, with a coating of fat. The same goes for the arms and legs. Weigh yourself before breakfast once a week, or more frequently if you like.

Inspirational Sayings

1. "Tough times pass, but tough people endure." — Schuller, Richard (2020).

This remark applies to all facets of life, but it is especially appreciated by professional lifters who push themselves to their ultimate limits. But especially as you begin weightlifting and training, there will be occasions when it isn't pleasurable, such as that last pull-up or barbell curl. After three sets of squats or splits, your thighs may be burning, and the last set of dumbbell rows may have you gasping for air. But after the set is over and the rest begins, the pain and burning sensation go away, and the workout always finishes with a sense of accomplishment, a sense of accomplishment. You're tough, and you're getting tougher.

2. "You must act like a champion to be a champion." — Luigi Ferrigno (2020).

Lou Ferrigno, the Incredible Hulk's champion weightlifter, contributed to this ideal mindset since he thinks that power comes from the inside. A championship attitude is inside all of us if we believe in ourselves and see the well-muscled, well-defined body we strive for. But it gets even better: if you want to be a well-built bodybuilder, you must train like one. Positive thinking is necessary to excite and inspire you, but it is useless without hard work and the commitment to give it your best.

3. "Don't want for it to be easier. "I wish you were stronger." Jim Rohm's (2020).

The concept causes us to believe that the workout, the lifting, and tugging, the squatting, and dipping, must be intense and difficult. This leads to the awareness that if something is simple, it is not done correctly. You must endeavor to stress your muscles to the degree where muscle cells and fibers are broken and must repair themselves through hypertrophy.

The awareness that it's a simple formula will propel you from passive to proactive: strength is directly proportionate to the effort invested in each session. Of course, a hard workout can be followed in two days by a less intense workout to aid recovery, but the next workout should be more intense. It will be worthwhile in the long run.

"It never gets any easier." You simply get stronger." — Not known (2020).

The goal is to gradually increase the weights until you can manage more without diminishing reps, sets, or rest intervals. For example, if you go to the dumbbell rack and take up a big weight, you can only complete one or two reps of a bicep curl. Do you wish you could perform more repetitions? Find a weight you can lift or curl for eight reps and have the patience and confidence to know that with discipline, you will progressively progress from the lesser weight to the higher weights and beyond.

Simply follow the standard method of lifting weights that max out at eight to ten reps, do three sets, and rest between sets and exercises.

5. "You must be at your strongest when you are at your weakest." — Not known (2020).

This motivation inspires weightlifters and cardio athletes to seek deep within the strength they know exists. Assume you are a runner preparing for a marathon or other long-distance competition. Even in the dead of winter, the only time you can train is early in the morning before work. At 5:30 a.m., you must get out of bed, wash your face, put on your running shoes, go outside, hit the road, and run into a searing cold headwind. What is it like to go through this every day for months? This is what inner power is all about, and it exemplifies, in the extreme, what someone chooses to do to achieve a goal. You will most likely not have to work out in such harsh conditions. You'll be inside, warm, lifting weights you can handle, and working to a schedule.

fair yet challenging effort peak but remember that runner in the dark, cold, early dawn, and let it inspire you to put in a stronger effort every day.

"Strength is not derived from physical capacity." It is the result of an unbreakable will." Gandhi, Mahatma (2020).

The strength and tenacity displayed by India's independence leader in calmly resisting overwhelming forces attest to the importance of resolve and devotion. Your willpower is what will enable you to achieve what others believe you are incapable of. To your friends, associates, and family, you may be wasting your time, putting yourself in danger, and for what? "You can't gain muscles at your age," they may say, or "It's too late for you."

Are they correct? The decision is entirely yours. If you have the desire and determination to commit to a consistent program of progressive weightlifting and aerobic exercise, you can grow muscle, get leaner and stronger, and improve your health, well-being, and lifespan.

"There are two kinds of pains: those that hurt you and those that transform you." — Not known (2020).

A weightlifter's point of view. Too much pain can be damaging, but when you need one more rep and the barbell feels like it weighs a ton, the ache of the extra effort you need now will pass, but your satisfaction will endure. Too much discomfort can be risky, resulting in injury and lowering your motivation to stick to the regimen. However, there is always some discomfort when attempting to hit your max production, and this is what you can expect and must suffer. The pain or strain you feel on the eighth or ninth rep will not harm you; you are lifting or pulling the appropriate weight for your ability at the time.

The pain you feel on the first or second rep indicates that the weight is too heavy for you and that you risk damage if you continue. Work gradually, and you will progress.

"Pain is only momentary." Quitting is permanent." Armstrong, Lance (2020).

The American Tour de France winner has braved cycling over the climbs of the Alps and Massif Central while fighting against the world's top cyclists. His determination, his drive, maintained him in the leader's yellow jersey for seven consecutive tours. While nothing will compare to the tribulation of a professional racer or weightlifter, you can learn from and be inspired by their example. The intensity of their training is almost unfathomable, and the harm they are doing to their bodies may have long-term implications. Don't try to emulate them, but let their "never quitting" attitude remind you on difficult days that you will forget the temporary pain, discomfort, or inconvenience, but you will be disappointed in yourself if you don't go the distance.

Can you come up with your own motivational and commitment quotations for muscle and strength building? All in all, you are the one who needs to be motivated, and no one understands you better than you. What makes you happy, enthusiastic, and energized?

Now for a change of pace. Let's step into the kitchen in Chapter 6 to learn how to eat better, healthier, and more satisfyingly to meet your bodybuilding and strength-building goals.

CHAPTER 6

Eating Well, (and Loving It)

Eating Well in Middle Age

One of the most underappreciated parts of physical health is the quality and composition of your nutrition. Many people believe they have done everything they can for their fitness and health by spending hours each week at the fitness center or home gym, and they believe this gives them permission to go into the kitchen and eat anything they want. This is not the case.

The cliché "you are what you eat" is true since your body can only digest and metabolize what you give it. As you can see, a healthy diet will benefit you in a variety of ways, from keeping you slimmer and helping you build muscles to providing you with the energy and stamina you need to get stronger and do more. Can a healthy diet help you live a longer life? Yes, because a good diet can help to delay or prevent the beginnings of heart disease, obesity, diabetes, chronic autoimmune illnesses, gastrointestinal problems, and degenerative diseases such as Alzheimer's.

Your Three Important Macronutrients

Macronutrients are defined by nutritionists as the three primary food groups we've discussed: carbs, proteins, and fats.

These are distinct from the numerous micronutrients such as vitamins and minerals. The macronutrients have been described on earlier pages, but for clarity, let's state the definitions here. They are named "macro" because they include the greater quantity of food we consume, as well as the total number of calories we consume, digest, assimilate, and metabolize.

"Macronutrients are the nutritive components of food that the body requires for energy and to sustain the body's structure and functions," says Lindsey Wolford, a wellness dietician at MD Anderson Cancer Center (2020).

The roles of macronutrients in energy, structure, and systems play are well defined

Carbohydrates are your body's principal fuel, providing energy for movement to your muscles and central nervous system, especially when the muscles are being pushed or exercised. According to Lindsey Wohlford, carbohydrates, or "carbs," should account for at least 45 percent and up to 65 percent of your daily calorie intake. Carbohydrates are found in grains and cereals, fruits and vegetables, and foods containing sugar and other sweeteners. There is a common misperception that carbohydrates are bad for us; yet, if they come from healthy sources like whole grains, fruits and vegetables, and nuts and seeds, they are the vital carbs your body requires to function. One gram of carbohydrates contains four calories.

Protein is required for the structure of your body, from muscles, ligaments, tendons, and bones to skin and hair, organs and nerves, cell membranes, and blood plasma.

All are composed of protein. Proteins govern the equilibrium of hormonal, enzyme, and metabolic systems.

In your body between acids and bases The RDA for protein is 0.8 grams per kilogram of body weight or 0.36 grams per pound, so a 150-pound person should consume roughly 50 grams of protein each day. When weightlifting to grow muscle, your daily protein consumption should be 75 grams or higher. One gram of protein contains four calories.

Protein sources in your diet are discussed in length later in this chapter.

Fats and oils (liquid fats at room temperature) are your body's concentrated energy store and contain more calories than the other two macronutrients. One gram of fat contains nine calories, making storage easier.

When carbs (stored in the muscles as glycogen) are low or exhausted, stored fats can be called upon for energy. Apart from producing energy, fats also aid in the insulation, protection, and cushioning of your organs, as well as the absorption and transport of fat-soluble nutrients such as vitamins D and E. The RDA for daily fat consumption is between 20% and 35% of total calories, with saturated fats accounting for no more than 10%. Monounsaturated and polyunsaturated fats from extra virgin olive oil, avocados, and vegetable oils from soybeans, sunflower, safflower, and corn are recommended to support cardiovascular health.

The Fitness and Weight Management 70:30 Rule

Is reaching a high level of physical fitness and maintaining a healthy weight due to 70% nutrition and 30% physical training? The notion that diet is more important than exercise has been popular among trainers and athletes for some time, but there does not appear to be a scientific basis for this specific ratio, though it appears to be trending in the right direction. There is scientific data that limits the amount of exercise that can contribute to weight loss.

According to the Guardian (2016), while exercise is unquestionably beneficial to your health and well-being, research reveals that physical activity alone will not necessarily burn more calories:

As a result, we can conclude that diet should be the primary weight-loss strategy.

This is based on research that shows that our metabolic processes reach a plateau beyond which more exercise, whether weightlifting, cardio, or combined, does not maintain the same rate of energy expenditure. After a certain point, the body adjusts to constrain, or limit, the number of calories burned at a certain time.

For example, after a day that includes a long, intense weightlifting and cardio activity that burned 650 more calories, your metabolism may slow down more than usual while resting and sleeping, resulting in a net calorie loss of only 150 to 250 calories. Other studies published in Current Biology (2016) involving humans and other primates found that those who engaged in extra physical activity did not burn significantly more calories in 24 hours than those who engaged in moderate activity, but both groups did burn more calories than sedentary individuals with low activity levels.

Professor Herman Panzer of the City University of New York, who took part in the study, stated, "Exercise is absolutely important."

"What our work adds is that we also need to focus on diet, particularly when it comes to managing our weight and avoiding or reversing harmful weight gain," they concluded (2016).

Diet is more important in maintaining a healthy weight and delivering the needed nutrients for muscle building, maintaining a healthy metabolism, regulating weight, and maintaining a robust immune system to keep disease and the ravages of aging at bay.

Your body's health and strength, as well as its energy and endurance, are all affected by the fuel you consume and the quality and types of meals you consume. As crucial as weightlifting is for muscle building and being stronger and more fit, your diet is equally, if not more, influential. Recognizing that our nutrition plays an important role in muscle building and fat loss, we'll help you cut through all the dietary misinformation and direct you to a lifelong dietary practice rather than a succession of fad diets that come and go. There are nutritional foundations that you will learn to follow.

Calories in versus calories out

It's called the CICO diet, but it's not a diet; it's a scientific principle. Calories In, Calories Out means that weight management is reliant on digesting the same number of calories that you expend each day. Because one pound of body weight contains 3,500 calories, if you want to lose one pound each week, you must consume 500 fewer calories than you burn each day of the week. The quantity you burn is determined by your metabolic rate, activity level, and what you have consumed, as certain foods are processed more easily and fully than others.

As you can see from the preceding section, exercise alone will not burn as many calories as you may imagine.

Reduce your calorie intake to enhance your CICO ratio.

A calorie is nothing more than a unit of energy. One gram of carbohydrate has four calories, and one gram of protein has four calories, but a gram of fat has nine calories, which is nature's effective means of storing energy and why diets high in fats and oils are, well, fatty.

Satiety: a sense of fullness

The satiety level of various foods is one of the ways they can be less or more fattening. The degree of fullness you experience lowers your hunger and desire to eat again. In general, protein-rich foods keep you fuller for longer because complex protein molecules are more difficult for your digestive system to break down into amino acid building blocks and then ingest. This contrasts with the simpler molecules that make up carbs and lipids, which pass through the stomach and are digested faster.

However, even items in the same category have varying amounts of satiety. A serving of boiling potatoes contains the same number of carbohydrates as a French pastry, such as a croissant, but the potatoes are seven times fuller, according to studies. This could be because the carbohydrates in potatoes are complex starches that take time to break down, whereas the croissant is built from two highly refined carbohydrates: white flour and sugar. It also contains butter, which is easily digestible.

The refined elements in the croissant highlight dietitians' concerns about overly refined and processed diets. Instead of focusing solely on calories, certified dietician Samantha Cassetti writes in Today (2020): "It's important to be aware of your calorie demands and to have an awareness of how calories from various foods make you feel." "Controlling your appetite," she says, "with filling foods that are also by your body's calorie needs is a good strategy to manage your weight and hunger levels."

Limiting Consumption of Highly Processed Foods

Highly processed foods account for around 60% of the average American diet and are blamed for introducing extra calories, sodium (salt), chemical additives (for preservation, flavor improvement, and color), saturated fats, and refined sugar. As a result, this diet causes weight gain, elevated LDL (bad) cholesterol levels, high blood pressure, and higher blood sugar levels.

A small-scale study published in Cell Metabolism (2019) illustrates the stark disparities between a diet high in processed meals and one high in complete, unprocessed foods.

Twenty participants first had a processed diet for two weeks before switching to natural, unprocessed, whole foods.

Both diets contained the same amount of carbohydrates, protein, fats and oils, and fiber. Importantly, individuals were free to consume as much or as little as they wished during the trial.

The following were the study's findings:

Participants on the processed diet consumed 500 calories per day more than those on the whole foods diet and gained two pounds.

The same people shed two pounds when they shifted to an unprocessed whole foods diet.

Participants ate faster and ate more during the processed diet phase, implying that the processed foods were less filling and signals of satiation were slower to reach the brain.

It is also plausible that higher levels of salt and flavor enhancers in processed foods encouraged faster and more frequent eating.

Conclusions include the fact that extra calories, regardless of source, lead to weight gain; additionally, it is hypothesized that unrefined, unprocessed meals, particularly grains, are slower to digest and absorb, potentially due to high fiber content, and also elevate resting metabolic rates.

Protein's Importance in Middle-Aged People

Our bodies require carbohydrates, protein, and lipids; however, as a middle-aged weightlifter striving to gain muscle mass, your demand for protein is greater than normal since you require that protein to create muscle tissue and allow hypertrophy to function successfully. Protein is even more important as you become older.

Protein offers distinct benefits for everyone, but notably for persons in their forties who desire to live an active lifestyle.

1. Loss of weight through appetite and hunger management.

Protein, as previously stated, digests more slowly than carbohydrates and fats.

Because it takes longer for stomach acids and enzymes to break it down, it remains in the stomach longer. Several hormonal variables influence weight:

Ghrelin is a hunger hormone that is inhibited by protein. This could be due to the protein digesting slowly, causing the stomach to send a signal to the brain to slow down ghrelin release as if to say, "full house, no room here."

Protein also stimulates the production of the hunger suppressor YY peptide. It fills you up and makes you less likely to grab something else to eat.

In a study of overweight women, participants raised their protein consumption from 15% to 30% and consumed 441 fewer calories per day on average. This could result in a one-pound decrease every eight days. The amount of protein required to meet 30% of a 2,000-calorie-per-day diet is 600 calories or 150 grams.

2. Reduced late-night snacking is another benefit of slow digesting protein and the appetite-suppressing effects of ghrelin and YY

peptides. A study of overweight men found that increasing protein consumption to 25% of total calories reduced late-night cravings.

Reduced by 60%, while the desire to snack at night was reduced by 50%

3. A muscle-building component. Protein is used to build muscle cells and fibers. During hypertrophy, when muscle cells and fibers are rebuilt after being damaged during a weightlifting workout, protein is the "brick and mortar" that is piled on and patched in. A lack of protein in the diet will slow hypertrophy and may result in muscle loss.

As a middle-aged weightlifter, you should be aware that your protein requirements are higher than those of people a decade or two younger. Your healing mechanisms and metabolism are slower, and you require more "raw materials" to restore the damaged protein in your muscles.

4. Protein is also required by bones. Age causes bone porosity, which leads to osteoporosis and the risk of broken bones.

While calcium is the most significant component of bones (and it is), protein also serves a crucial role in helping to reinforce the calcium, making the bones stronger and less porous. This disproves the myth that protein weakens bones by leaching calcium away; this is just not true.

5. Increased metabolism and fat burning Eating and the digesting process burn calories and fat because labor is done and energy is expended. This is known as the thermic effect of food, and it varies based on the type of food being digested. Protein has a four times larger thermic effect than carbohydrates or lipids, thus it improves metabolism and burns more calories. In one study, the higher protein diet burnt roughly 100 more calories, and in another study that

compared a high-protein group to a low-protein group, the high protein group had a net caloric burn of 260 calories per day.

6. Aids in the prevention of heart disease. An analysis of 40 separate research on increased protein in the diet discovered that systolic blood pressure (top number) was reduced by 1.76 mm Hg and diastolic blood pressure (bottom, smaller number) was reduced by 1.76 mm Hg.

By 1.15 millimeters of mercury LDL (bad), cholesterol and triglycerides were also reduced. These findings imply that consuming more protein may help avoid strokes, heart attacks, and chronic kidney disease.

7. Improves recuperation time after an injury. When you are hurt, the majority of the damage is done to your skeletal muscles, which are formed of protein and require protein to repair themselves. Protein is required for bone healing.

A higher protein diet also increases platelets in the blood, which are responsible for clotting and stopping bleeding.

Maintaining fitness as you get older. Muscular weakness and loss of muscle mass are inevitable consequences of aging. Increased protein in the diet combined with resistance exercises has been shown to prevent the beginning of sarcopenia, which is age-related muscle loss and degradation. The exercise will promote muscle growth and regeneration, but enough protein levels are required for hypertrophy to function properly.

Protein Sources

The following foods are high in protein and provide additional muscle-building and health advantages. We start with dairy and egg protein sources, then go on to fish and seafood, meat, and plant protein sources.

Protein Sources from Dairy and Eggs

Greek yogurt contains more protein than regular yogurt because it is strained to eliminate some of the water, concentrating on what remains. A 34-cup serving has 16 to 19 grams of protein, which is double that of normal yogurt. Greek yogurt has both fast-digesting whey protein and slow-digesting casein protein. The live probiotic bacteria cultures, which nourish the microbiome in the gut, provide additional benefits. High-protein Greek yogurt is also available in Icelandic and Australian varieties. Check the labels to ensure that the protein content is correct. To reduce calories and avoid saturated fats, choose low-fat or fat-free alternatives.

Milk is a healthy source of protein and carbs, and whole milk can contain up to 4% partly saturated fat, there are plenty of low-fat and fat-free options available (and recommended vs. full fat). Milk, like yogurt, has both quick and slow digesting proteins, which are thought to help with muscle growth and muscle cell and fiber improvement. According to studies, drinking milk after a hard workout results in more muscle gain than the same exertion followed by carbohydrates.

Cottage cheese is a high-protein food, with 28 grams in a one-cup, eight-ounce dose. Cottage cheese protein, like other dairy protein sources, is high in the muscle-building amino acid leucine. Like milk and dairy, you can get fat-free, low-fat, or full-fat versions. Because dairy fats are high in saturated fats, you should choose fat-free or low-fat alternatives.

Eggs are high in protein, with one egg comprising six grams and only 70 calories. Eggs are abundant in leucine, an amino acid that is essential for muscular growth. Even though eggs contain cholesterol, they have extra nutritional benefits such as choline and B vitamins and should be consumed. Increase you're if you prefer.

Protein Sources from Fish and Seafood

Salmon is a cold-water fish strong in omega-3 fatty acids, which have antioxidant properties and are thought to aid in muscle building. A six-ounce meal of lean salmon steak contains 34 grams of protein. Canned salmon is high in protein and minerals as well. Other Coldwater fish such as cod, sea bass, turbot, mackerel, and sardines are also advised, as is tuna, which will be mentioned later.

Tuna has even more protein than salmon, with 40 grams in a six-ounce portion, as well as vitamin A and B vitamins including B6, B12, and niacin, all of which help with energy and workout performance. Tuna also has a high concentration of antioxidant omega-3 acids, which are thought to reduce the incidence of age-related muscle loss. Canned tuna, like salmon, is high in protein and nutrients when compared to fresh.

Shrimp, with 36 grams of protein in a six-ounce serving, is another high-protein seafood option. Shrimp contain a high concentration of the muscle-building amino acid leucine. A six-ounce dish of shrimp comprises only 144 calories and contains almost no carbs.

Scallops have a similar nutritional profile as shrimp, but are heavier in calories and protein, with 40 grams in a six-ounce portion.

Protein Sources from Meat

Chicken breast, served lean with the skin removed and any visible fat removed, is high in protein, with 26 grams in a three-ounce meal and 52 grams in a six-ounce piece. There are also adequate doses of vitamins B6 and niacin, which are associated with assisting your body's performance during exercise and promoting muscular growth.

Lean beef is similar to chicken breast in terms of protein content, but the issue is finding beef that is low in fat. Choose a lean steak and trim away any visible fat to avoid fatty cuts. Avoid cuts that are marbled with unremovable fat. When using ground beef, choose 95 percent lean, which has fewer saturated fat calories: a three-ounce portion of 95 percent lean beef has 145 calories, compared to 228 calories for 70 percent lean beef.

Turkey breast is an extremely lean white meat that has 25 grams of protein per three-ounce portion when served without the skin (which may have a layer of fat). This serving's 100 calories are almost entirely fat and carbohydrate-free, and it's abundant in muscle-building B vitamins, including niacin, like chicken breast.

Plant Protein Sources

There are a few plant-based foods that include a complete protein with all nine necessary amino acids that we require in our diets, but most plant sources are insufficient and must be supplemented with complementary plant-based meals:

Beans, legumes, and grains supply all of the amino acids required for nutritionally complete protein.

A meal made with black, pinto, or kidney beans and brown rice or wheat-based pasta, for example, delivers nutritionally complete protein.

When compared to plant-sourced protein, protein levels in animal-derived foods are significantly more concentrated and deliver more protein per ounce or measure.

For good reason, soybeans are the most well-known plant source of complete protein. 12 cup cooked soybeans contain 14 grams of protein, as well as healthy unsaturated fats, vitamin K, and the minerals iron and phosphorus.

You can also select immature fresh or frozen soybeans known as edamame. Edamame beans have 17 grams of protein and eight grams of fiber, which improves digestion. It includes high levels of manganese and vitamin K, as well as folate, which has been linked to improved amino acid processing and muscular building in middle-aged and older persons.

Quinoa is a grain that contains whole or nearly complete protein as well as a significant amount of unrefined, nutritious carbs for energy. One cup of cooked quinoa provides eight grams of protein, 40 grams of carbohydrates, and five grams of fiber to aid digestion. It contains phosphorus and magnesium, which aid in the coordination of the neurological system with skeletal muscles.

Beans, such as kidney, lima, black, and pinto, are high in vegetative-source protein, with 15 grams in one cup of cooked beans. Beans, as previously stated, require to go with grains and cereals such as rice, oats, quinoa, wheat, and rye (in bread or pasta, for example). Beans are high in nutrients such as B vitamins and minerals such as iron, phosphorus, and magnesium.

Brown rice, oats, chickpeas, peanuts, almonds, and buckwheat (used in baking instead of flour) are other protein-rich plant foods. Grains and grains provide less protein and more cars than beans and legumes. Nuts have more unsaturated and healthy oils than other foods, but they are high in calories, so limit your intake.

Is There a Perfect Diet?

Enter a bookshop and browse for the diet books area. You'll need time only to read the titles because there are so many diets offered. There are various causes for this, including:

Many people require assistance and direction to lose weight and manage ailments and illnesses such as diabetes, heart disease, hypertension, cancer, immunological disorders, and psychological problems, among others.

There is a widespread misconception that there is a miracle diet, a one-size-fits-all answer to losing weight, building muscle, curing sickness, and living longer.

Diet is all about eating, and as indicated by the size of the cookbook area at the bookshop, people take food extremely seriously.

Let's take a quick look at some of the popular diets today, but keep in mind that while there are reasonable ways to aid with weight control and avoid or alleviate certain ailments, there is no single fantastic diet that is the solution to everyone's issues. There is no such thing as a "one-size-fits-all" death because every one of us has our physiology, metabolic rate, and sensitivities.

Popular diets

Fasting has recently surfaced as a means to better health, happiness, and longer life, but you should be aware that while research on worms and mice has been promising, studies on humans are primarily in the early phases. The more common ways are intermittent fasting, which is done on a daily, repeated basis, such as the 16:8 fasting diet, which allows eating for eight hours (e.g., 8 a.m. to 4 p.m.) and then nothing for the next sixteen hours (4 p.m. to 8 a.m.). There are harsher variants, such as 18:6. Some people experiment with prolonged fasting, going for 24- or even 48-hour fasts followed by a day of unrestrained food. People who do this tend not to overeat on non-fast days since their stomachs shrink slightly during the fast.

Fasting diets can help you grow muscle as a weightlifter.

Are not recommended for you.

Paleo diets trace back to simpler times when our forefathers were hunter-gatherers and ate "off the land," which meant anything they could find. This motivates diets today that avoid all refined and processed foods (which is admirable) and are based on foods that our bodies evolved to digest successfully over millions of years.

According to the Mayo Clinic, a paleo diet often consists of vegetables, fruits, nuts and seeds, lean meats, and fish, all of which can be obtained by hunting and gathering. A paleo diet restricts dairy products, grains and legumes, and potatoes, which became available around 10,000 years ago when cultivation and agriculture began. Additional salt is also avoided. Overall, the paleo diet is considered healthy and wholesome as long as macronutrient ratios are followed and a variety of foods are consumed to ensure enough levels of vitamins and minerals are consumed.

The keto diet, short for ketogenic, has a very particular goal: quick weight loss by stimulating fat burning.

This is accomplished by eating a high-fat, low-carbohydrate diet, basically substituting carbs with fats. This

This causes a metabolic condition known as ketosis, which is highly efficient in utilizing stored and ingested fat for energy instead of carbs and glycogen. You lose weight by burning fat.

Another characteristic is the conversion of fat stored in the liver to ketones, which provide energy to the brain. Furthermore, the keto diet has been demonstrated to lower blood sugar and insulin levels, which may help to prevent or reduce diabetes and other illnesses. Other advantages include a sense of fullness (satiety), which lessens desires to eat or snack, and an enhanced mood. Long-term implications of keto and other very low-carb diets are being studied.

While the keto diet looks to be beneficial for weight loss, it may not provide enough protein for muscle building; at least 30% of your meal should include protein.

The Mediterranean diet Let us conclude with a diet that is not only gaining widespread acceptance but is also the most similar to the perfect diet that everyone is looking for. It comprises a large variety of delicious foods, is inexpensive, is regarded as heart-healthy by the medical profession, and may help slow the onset of many other ailments, ranging from diabetes to cancer.

This diet is based on the behaviors of long-term Mediterranean Basin residents, including areas of Italy, Spain, and France, who live healthier, longer lives. But, more importantly, these people adopt a lifestyle that includes not only diet, but also being physically active throughout their lives, maintaining a healthy weight, and maintaining a happy outlook on life.

The Mediterranean diet includes the following components: A variety of fresh vegetables, fresh and dried fruits, nuts and seeds, whole grains and cereals, fish, lean meat in modest servings (e.g., six ounces), moderate amounts of dairy (mainly as cheese), eggs, extra virgin olive oil, and moderate amounts of red wine.

Whatever diet you choose, keep in mind that as a weightlifter and muscle builder, you need enough protein in your diet and should eat foods low in saturated fats. Avoid salty foods, processed foods, fried foods, and anything high in sugar. The next section discusses both good and harmful food sources.

Good and Bad Food Sources

The types and sources of the three macronutrients have been thoroughly addressed, but here is a summary of the good and bad. While this chapter has been devoted to assisting you in understanding the meals that are best for your health and improving your level of physical fitness, building muscle, and making you stronger, there are carbohydrate, protein, and fat sources that you should avoid. We've listed both the approved sources of your macronutrients and the items that have been identified as undesired and potentially dangerous to help you plan your diet.

Nutritionists at MD Anderson Cancer Center say:

Dairy products, such as milk, yogurt, and cottage cheese, are recommended carbohydrate sources, with a preference for low-fat or non-fat because full-fat dairy products are rich in saturated fats and calories. Nondairy replacements derived from soy, almonds, and oats are also high in carbohydrates. Dairy products are also a good source of complete protein.

Vegetables, which are low in calories and high in vitamins and minerals, can be consumed without restriction.

Choose a variety of colors (green, yellow, red, and purple) to supply a variety of micronutrients.

Fruits are high in natural sugars (thus their sweetness) and micronutrients. Fruit should be consumed without the extra sugar and in its natural, solid shape to preserve the pulp, which contains important fiber. Many juices include sugar and have had the pulp removed.

Legumes, which include beans, peas, and lentils, are abundant in carbs, fiber, and many of the 20 amino acids that make up protein.

Whole grains, such as whole wheat, rye, buckwheat, spelled, corn, and oats, are high in carbohydrates and high in fiber.

Vitamin B and fiber sources These extra properties are not present in refined grains.

Avoid refined flours and sugar, which can be found in crackers, most bread, cookies, and breakfast cereals, and sugar, which can be found in most fruit juices, soft drinks, athletic performance beverages, and candies.

Beans, particularly black, pinto, and kidney beans, as well as lentils and soy products, are recommended protein sources. Except for soy, the proteins are deficient and must be supplemented with grains and cereals.

Nuts and seeds, including sugar-free nut butter.

Whole grains such as quinoa, rye, wheat, spelled, corn, and soy are acceptable, with the caveat that the amino acids do not constitute full protein.

Meat, poultry, fish and seafood, dairy, and eggs are all sources of animal protein.

Avoid processed meats such as sausages, salami, bacon, frankfurters (hot dogs), and canned lunch meats.

Lean red meat consumption should be limited to 18 ounces per week.

Vegetable oils, particularly extra virgin olive oil, avocado oil, and canola oil, are recommended fat sources, as are oils derived from corn, sunflower, and safflower.

Cold-water salmon, tuna, mackerel, and sardines are examples of fatty fish.

Flax seeds, chia seeds, avocados, and olives are all good sources of omega-3 fatty acids.

Nuts and seeds, as well as natural nut butter with no added sugar.

Avoid these fat sources:

Fried foods are created with refined flour and absorb a lot of trans-fat-containing oils.

Animal sources include full-fat dairy products such as milk, butter, yogurt, and cream cheese, as well as the fats found in meats and fowl.

Coconut and palm oils, shortening (used in baking), soft tub margarine, and the majority of packaged baked items (read the labels for fat content).

Now, on to Chapter 7 and dispelling some popular myths about working out, getting in shape, creating muscles, and gaining power after the age of 40.

CHAPTER 7

Common Fitness After 40 Misconceptions

What should I believe? You're in your forties and preparing to embark on a serious strengthening and fitness regimen. Is it secure? Is this something you should be doing at your age? Perhaps you've been cautioned by others or have your concerns. Let's get down to business.

1. You're too old to lift weights and run a marathon.

Let's put this myth to rest as soon as possible. There is no age restriction for getting in shape. If you are 40, 50, or 60 years old, male or female, you need a decent workout regimen now more than ever. Yes, it would have been easier if you had the muscles and arteries of a 20-year-old, but your body took care of itself back then. Your metabolism is now slower, fat accumulates more quickly, and you are losing muscle mass. Your bones may be becoming more porous and prone to fracture. A good resistance and aerobics program can cure these aging effects. If you're new to this and out of shape, consult your doctor first, as we recommend in Chapter 4, to receive the right precautions, and then start to work on restoring your body's fitness and health potential.

2. You should devote more time to exercise.

Being in your forties is not an excuse to increase your training time. When it comes to an intensive, quality workout, less is more, so there's no reason to overdo it or waste time that could be spent elsewhere. Even if time does not allow for a full workout at the gym, you may still spend 20 minutes at home working out with weights or practicing bodyweight calisthenics. Even if there is no time constraint, full weightlifting or cardiovascular workout can be completed in 40 minutes or less. Any more may result in overwork injuries.

Control your schedule to enhance your training, especially in middle age.

3. Avoid doing high-intensity workouts.

It all depends on your definition of intensity. Weightlifting has overwhelming proof that you can gain muscle in your forties if you progressively work up to your peak levels and discover the sweet spot between too little and too much weight. Here's a recap of the book's suggestions. After warming up, execute eight to ten reps with weights that you can only make the last one or two reps with. If you can't do more than eight, it's too heavy, and if you can do more than ten, it's too light. Do three sets of eight to ten reps with the appropriate weight, and your workout will be intense enough.

4. You don't have time to exercise.

Maybe you're at a point in your job where everything is on the line and you need to arrive early and stay late. You believe that taking 30 or 40 minutes out of your day is simply not feasible.

Remembering Parkinson's law, which states that labor expands to fill the available time, you should reconsider your work ethic; you may discover that you have more free time. Ask yourself if you truly lack the time or if you lack the passion to exercise, get stronger, and be fit. If you skipped through to this chapter instead of reading the book, go back to Chapter 5 and read about motivation and commitment. You may also break up your workouts by getting up and moving about for a few minutes here and there during the day. Short bursts of activity can burn calories, challenge muscles, and strengthen the heart, according to research.

Running is risky and should be avoided.

Running in your forties carries some risks. We need to determine the best, safe approach to run, especially for your joints and connective tissues. Ideally, you should run on a treadmill, which softens your steps and is less likely to cause knee pain.

which are the most prone to wear and strain as time passes If you must run outside, use softer surfaces such as grass or pathways through forests and parks. Wear a nice pair of running shoes to cushion your foot and prevent it from rolling. If running gets too painful, consider switching to race walking, which is less strenuous on the joints while still providing an excellent cardio workout.

6. You don't need to perform both diet and exercise to lose weight.

This is covered in Chapter 6, but to summarize: nutrition is by far the most influential in weight management.

The prevailing scientific premise is calories in, calories out (how many calories you digest vs. how many you burn), and it is considerably simpler to avoid eating the 500calorie pair of iced doughnuts or a cup of full-fat ice cream than it is to run or walk five miles to burn those calories off. Especially when studies show that calories burnt during activity are largely countered by a slower metabolism while resting or sleeping. The easiest strategy to lose weight is to eat less and maintain a reasonable diet (not a fad diet) while continuing your fitness regimen. Increase your protein intake to help strengthen muscles, keep you satisfied for longer, and make you less prone to snacks.

7. It's too late to get rid of tummy fat.

The same "calories in, calories out" rule applies here. If you burn more calories in a given period than you ingest and digest, you will lose weight and excess fat. True, as you become older and your metabolism slows, the fat tends to build around your belly. Even if you maintain a good caloric deficit, that fat won't last long. Unfortunately, we cannot "spot decrease" fat, which means that abdominal exercises such as leg raises and planks will tighten the muscles but have little effect on belly fat. If you want to lose fat, the greatest way to do so is with a combination of food and exercise.

CONCLUSION

This book was prepared for anyone over the age of 40 who is thinking about getting into good physical shape for the first time or returning to the good shape they had when they were younger. If you're worried that it's too late for you, that you've waited too long to start or continue working out, this book will reassure you that it's not too late. Your timing is perfect.

Let us summarize the main points of the book.

Has been covered

Your body has changed. Your physique is no longer that of a 20-year-old or even a 30-year-old; your metabolism is slowing, subtly but progressively, year after year, and you've been losing muscle mass and gaining fat. These changes might be noticeable or subtle, but they are a normal part of the aging process. These changes, however, are not unavoidable and can be slowed, stopped, or even reversed with a well-planned fitness program that includes weightlifting and other resistance exercises, cardiovascular training, and a healthy diet.

Are you stronger after 40? Can you gain muscle and strength after the age of 40? Yes, because there is science behind sweat, exertion, and training. It's called hypertrophy, and it refers to the process of ripping down muscle cells and fiber when lifting weights, then resting while your body repairs the damage by adding protein and slightly overbuilds. Overbuilding develops over time, resulting in larger, stronger muscles. This process may be slower at 40 or 50, but it occurs regardless.

You can work out hard, just not in the same way.

Once you understand how to perform the appropriate exercises with the right weights and routines, your age is no longer an impediment to gaining serious muscular bulk and definition.

Heavy weight lifting When it comes to deciding how much weight to lift safely and successfully, the alternatives range from numerous reps of light weights to very few — one, two, or three — reps that you can barely handle. The best weights are those that you can lift eight to ten times with the last rep being extremely difficult to lift, pull, or push all the way. So, yes, you can lift high weights if you stick to the eight-to-ten reps maximum.

Motivation, dedication, and consistency A good muscle-building, strength, and fitness program demand motivation to begin, but perhaps more crucially, an unwavering determination to renew your devotion to weightlifting and cardiovascular training over time:

Without motivation, you may procrastinate indefinitely or begin your workouts half-heartedly. However, enthusiasm is only a spark to get you started; commitment and consistency will drive you to attain your muscle-building and fitness goals. You may be tempted to quit or slow down in your progressive training if you are not committed and consistent, and this will not get you where you need to go.

Begin each day with a vision of whom you want to be.

Consider those stronger biceps, the well-defined chest and abdominals, the strong legs, and the flat stomach. Commit yourself every morning, as soon as you get up, to acquire that body, that power, vitality, and energy.

Consistency necessitates willpower, something you are well aware of. You can rely on it every day to put on those gym shorts and workout shoes and give your muscles and heart the conditioning they require and deserve as you renew your effort and dedication to longevity and health.

Consider each workout to be a long-term physical equity investment. Hypertrophy, like building a solid wall a few bricks and mortar at a time, gradually but steadily grows muscle tissue. Make a long-term commitment to growth.

In middle age, progress may be slow and undetectable on a daily or weekly basis, but by making your workouts a consistent routine over the months and years, your dedication to consistency will pay off with the body you desire. Slow progress is preferable to no progress, and with persistence and patience, great results will be yours.

Your workouts may vary in intensity, and some days will be more gratifying than others. But there are no terrible workouts; all that is required is that you show up because the only "poor" workout is the one you don't perform. Remember the tip: on days when it's difficult to even think about working out, tell yourself you'll simply do a few dumbbell lifts and push-ups, but that once you get started and warmed up, your energy will return and you'll put in a good workout.

You've got this. This book will show you how to get started and keep your commitment and resolve to achieve your muscle, strength, and fitness goals. You've seen celebrity athletes' routines, from James Bond to The Rock, and while you probably won't follow their extreme regimens, you can be inspired by their dedication and discipline.

Do not cause any harm. You have noted the upfront warning of not harming and being mindful of your age and body when offering a variety of weightlifting workouts and calisthenics.

Warm-up and begin cautiously with lighter weights until you get the hang of it.

Where should I work out? You might have access to a well-equipped health club, fitness center, or gym.

For cardiovascular training, utilize free weights, exercise machines with cables to pull and handles to push, as well as rubber stretch bands (which may simulate many weight and machine actions), and treadmill and elliptical machines. You could also want a home gym with free weights, such as dumbbells and barbells.

Rubber stretches bands and tubes, as well as a pull-up and a chin-up bar

Bodyweight calisthenics is another wonderful alternative that requires absolutely no equipment and can be done at home or anyplace. Think about how much weight you're lifting when you do push-ups, squats, or pull-ups; your body weight can create a lot of resistance.

Work out your entire body. The seven weightlifting and seven calisthenics movements are more than enough to give you a full-body workout that works every muscle group. If you have access to weights, you should incorporate routines from both categories;

otherwise, bodyweight calisthenics can produce equally amazing results. Each exercise contains a link to a video demonstration with clear instructions from expert trainers, allowing you to learn and practice the exercises safely and effectively.

Rest and recuperation You've been said that rest and recovery are essential since the process of hypertrophy takes time, and it takes much longer as you get older. Between resistance workouts, muscle groups should rest for at least one day, preferably two. You can work out the entire body and then recover for two or three days, or you can work out more frequently and limit each workout to one or two muscle groups, such as arms and shoulders on Monday, chest, and core on Tuesday, legs on Wednesday, and back to arms and shoulders on Thursday. You can choose the routines and times that work best for you. Each muscle group should be worked at least twice a week.

The metabolic rate. You've been briefed on your metabolism to understand what it is, how it affects your bodily functions, and why and how it slows as you get older. The need of being highly motivated to begin your strengthening and fitness program is underlined once more, as is the requirement for long-term commitment to keep your fitness program going and make it a cherished component of your daily. Hopefully, the motivational quotations in that section can boost your motivation.

You are what you consume. The topic of diet was thoroughly explored, to clarify the sometimes-misunderstood role of carbohydrates, proteins, and fats — the macronutrients — in providing our bodies with energy, structure, and function. CICO, or the concept of calories in, and calories out, makes it clear that if you want to lose weight, you must consume fewer calories than you expend each day.

The importance of protein for weightlifters and exercise aficionados in their forties is discussed, and a list of recommended sources of healthy protein from both animal and plant sources is provided.

Various popular diets were discussed, and you are recommended to follow a diet like the Mediterranean, which encourages a wide variety of fruits and vegetables, lean meat and fish, grains, beans and cereals, nuts and seeds, olive oil, and even red wine in moderation.

Those who adhere to this diet eat for pleasure as well as health and fitness, and they lead an active lifestyle.

Misconceptions about exercise. We closed by dispelling some common myths about weightlifting and training after the age of 40 and providing reassurance that, yes, you can and should stay healthier, stronger, less prone to sustain injuries and help avoid diseases. Despite your hectic schedule, you have the time to exercise and should lift big weights. Maintaining a healthy weight requires both nutrition and activity, and yes, you can burn fat at your age.

Let's get started. What are you waiting for if you haven't started your strengthening and fitness program yet? To summarize, I would say: " "The ideal day to begin was yesterday. Now is the second-best time."

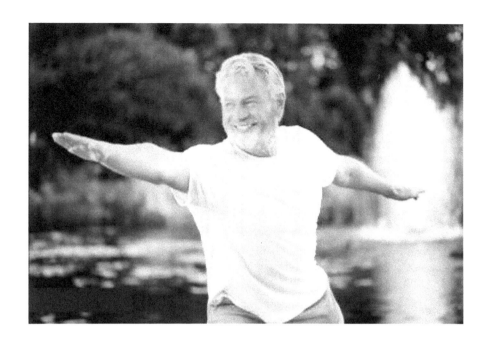

CPSIA information can be obtained
at www.ICGtesting.com
Printed in the USA
BVHW031440131022
649370BV00010B/749